Growing GREEN InterActions—Wise Action Tools

A Social Literacy Program to Be Our Better Selves in a Better World

Herb Hein, MMSc, CCC-SLP

Hein SLP, Inc. San Diego, California

Growing G.R.E.E.N. InterActions—*Wise Action Tools*

A Social Literacy Program to Be Our Better Selves in a Better World

Published by Hein SLP, Inc. San Diego, California

www.HeinSLPinc.com

Permissions, requests, and correspondence should be directed to the publisher.

ISBN-13: 978-0-9659878-2-0

This first edition printed in the United States of America.

Wise Action Tools

1. G.R.E.E.N. Token Tracker
2. Who Is on a Team with You?
3. Our Common Team Goals
4. G.R.E.E.N. Actions Evaluation Chart
5. G.R.E.E.N. Action Report
6. My Personal G.R.E.E.N. Action Tracker
7. Classroom Team G.R.E.E.N. Action Tracker
8. Home Team G.R.E.E.N. Action Tracker
9. Work Team G.R.E.E.N. Action Tracker
10. Our Classroom Team Rules
11. Our Home Team Rules
12. Our Friendship Team Rules
13. Our Work Team Rules
14. Self-Check: Are You Making Your Best Life Story? (2 pages)
15. Picture Your Own Best Life!
16. My Personal Goal Worksheet
17. Noting Progress on My Personal Goals
18. Ready, Set, Goal! My Goal for Right Now
19. I Draw Myself Using a Guiding G.R.E.E.N. Thought
20. Guiding G.R.E.E.N. Thought Memory Challenge
21. Civilized Choice Checker

G.R.E.E.N. Token Tracker

I AM CIVILIZED & G.R.E.E.N.

G rateful	**Grateful**—I appreciate what I have
R espectful	**Respectful**—I am polite and well mannered
E mpathetic	**Empathetic**—I care about the feelings of others
E asygoing	**Easygoing**—I am cooperative
N avigating	**Navigating**—I use strategies to cope with challenges

Growing G.R.E.E.N. InterActions® HeinSLP, Inc. www.heinslpinc.com

G.R.E.E.N. Token Tracker

I AM CIVILIZED & G.R.E.E.N.

G rateful	**Grateful**—I appreciate what I have
R espectful	**Respectful**—I am polite and well mannered
E mpathetic	**Empathetic**—I care about the feelings of others
E asygoing	**Easygoing**—I am cooperative
N avigating	**Navigating**—I use strategies to cope with challenges

Growing G.R.E.E.N. InterActions® HeinSLP, Inc. www.heinslpinc.com

Wise Action Tool #1

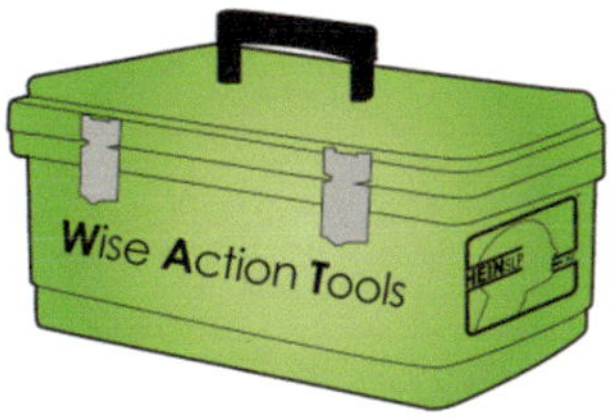

WHO IS ON A TEAM WITH YOU?

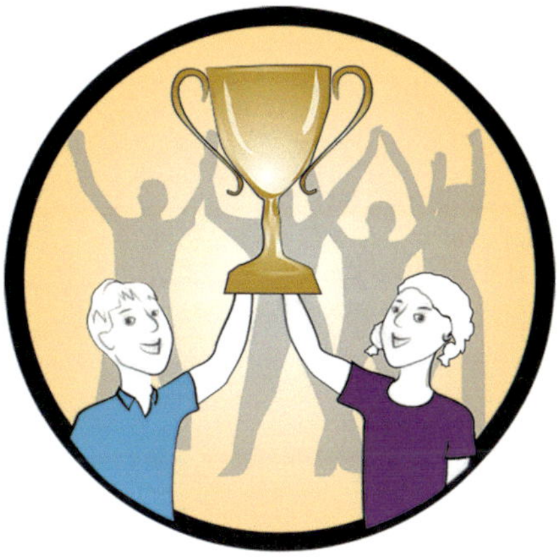

You make the world better when you think of other people. in addition to yourself. You can be more **civil** and help your part of civilization be more civilized! You have more **power** when you realize that you and the people around you are all on the same Team!

Who is on your Team? Who else should you be thinking about besides yourself?

What are your **powerful** Teams? If you are a member of a Team, check it off to show you are part of it. Add any other Teams that you might be on if they are not listed already:

______ Home Team (parents, siblings, children)

______ Classroom Team (teacher, aides, therapists, classmates, students)

______ Friendship Team (old friends, new friends, future friends)

______ Sports Team (coaches, teammates, umpires, referees)

______ Work Team (boss, coworkers)

______ ____

______ ____

Wise Action Tool #2

Wise Action Tools

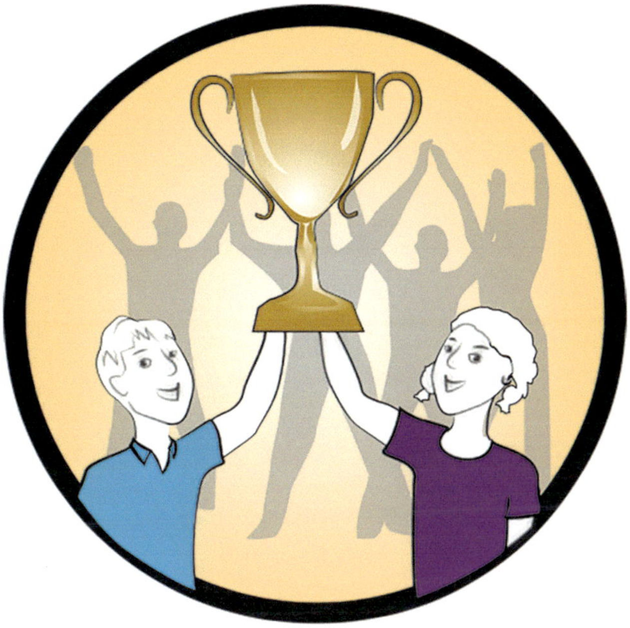

OUR TEAM NAME ______________________________

OUR COMMON TEAM GOALS

____

____

____

____

____

____

Wise Action Tool #3

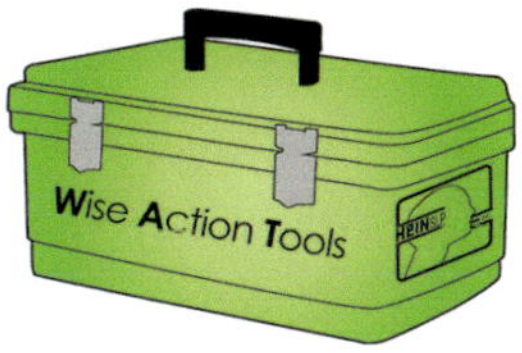

G.R.E.E.N. ACTIONS EVALUATION CHART

Team Member ______________________ Today's Date ______________________

Evaluation by:

- ☐ Self
- ☐ Teacher
- ☐ Parent
- ☐ Peer
- ☐ Other ______________

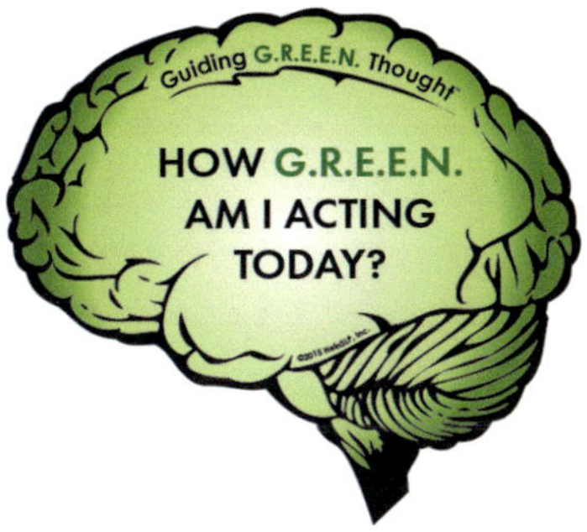

HONESTLY EVALUATION ACTIONS BY CHECKING THE BOX THAT IS TRUE TODAY

	NEVER 0	A LITTLE BIT 1	HALF THE TIME 2	MOST OF THE TIME 3	ALL THE TIME 4	TOTAL
GRATEFUL—I let people know that I appreciate what I have.						
RESPECTFUL—I am respectful of the people and things in every situation. I use a tone of voice that is positive and polite.						
EMPATHETIC—I show that I am considerate of the feelings of my friends, classmates, and family.						
EASYGOING—I am open-minded and cooperate with people to meet Team Goals.						
NAVIGATING—I am flexible when I manage challenges because I stay calm and make wise choices.						
I take responsibility for my actions and accept consequences.						
				GRAND TOTAL		

Wise Action Tool #4

G.R.E.E.N. ACTION REPORT

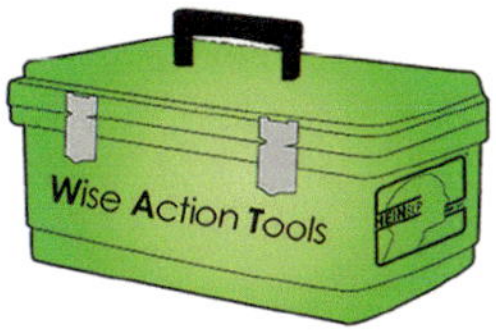

Date: ____________________ Situation: ____________________

____

____

Who acted **G.R.E.E.N.**? ____

Circle the behavior(s) shown:

Grateful **R**espectful **E**mpathetic **E**asygoing **N**avigating

What was the **G.R.E.E.N.** action? ______________________________

____

____

GROWING G.R.E.E.N. InterActions™

G.R.E.E.N. ACTION REPORT

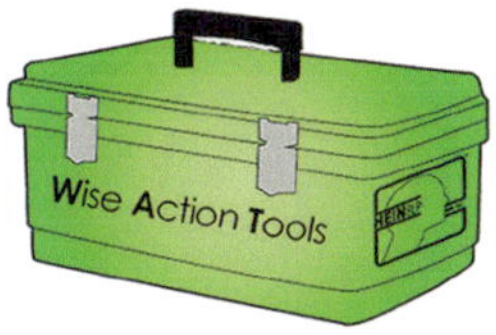

Date: ____________________ Situation: ____________________

____

____

Who acted **G.R.E.E.N.**? ____

Circle the behavior(s) shown:

Grateful **R**espectful **E**mpathetic **E**asygoing **N**avigating

What was the **G.R.E.E.N.** action? ______________________________

____

____

GROWING G.R.E.E.N. InterActions™ **©HeinSLP, INC.**

Wise Action Tool #5

MY NAME ______________________________

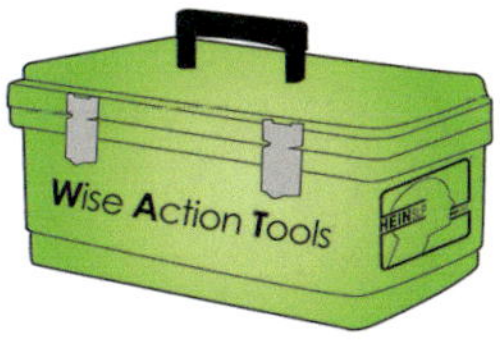

MY PERSONAL G.R.E.E.N. ACTION TRACKER

How many times can I act G.R.E.E.N. this week?

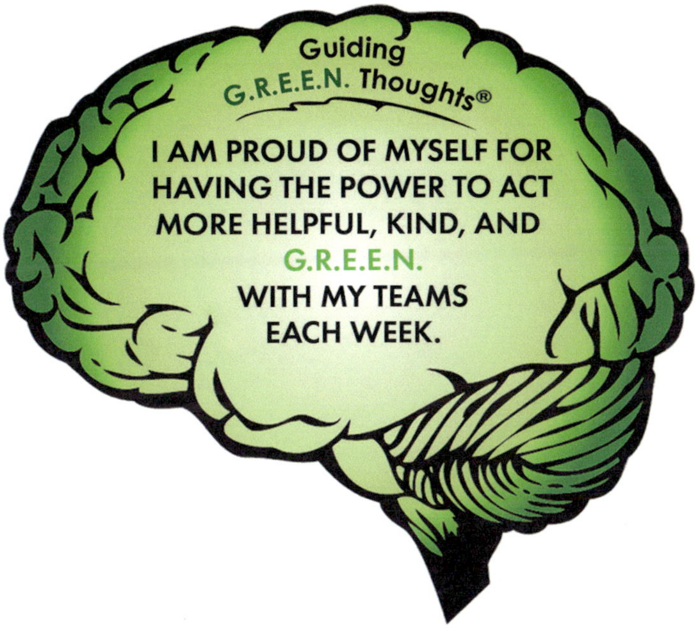

I am acting G.R.E.E.N. when I take action that others think is caring, civil, cooperative, considerate, easygoing, empathetic, grateful, helpful, kind, navigating, polite, positive, respectful, supportive, or thoughtful. When others on my Teams notice me acting G.R.E.E.N. and give me a G.R.E.E.N. **Action Report**, I put a check mark in the box for that day. I also can fill out a G.R.E.E.N. **Action Report** for myself when I notice that I have acted G.R.E.E.N.with someone, and I can then give myself a check mark in the box for that day.

I see how many times I can act G.R.E.E.N. this week.
Then I can see if I can act G.R.E.E.N. even more times next week!

Date	Date	Date	Date	Date	Date	Date

This week's G.R.E.E.N. Action Total: ____________

Wise Action Tool #6

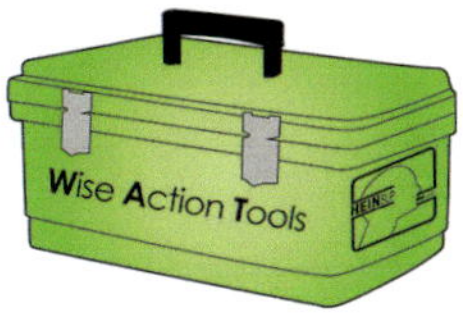

CLASSROOM TEAM G.R.E.E.N. ACTION TRACKER

Name of our Classroom Team: ______________________________

This is our Team Action Tracker for the week starting on ________________
(date)

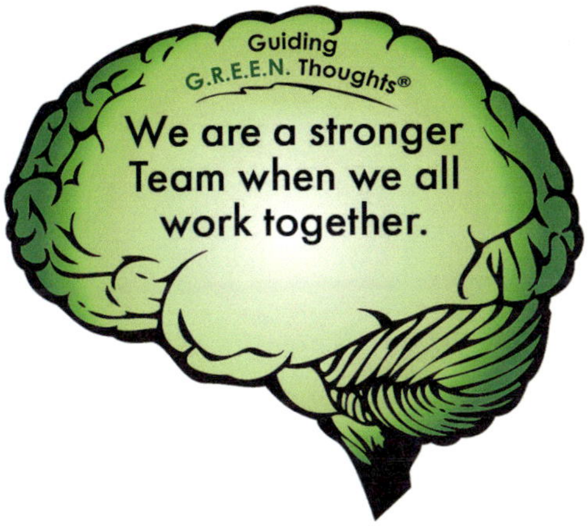

Fill in the names of everyone on the Team.

√ Check the box under the date each time a Classroom Team member acted G.R.E.E.N. or transfer the total from each Team member's **Personal G.R.E.E.N. Action Tracker.**

Classroom Teammates	Monday	Tuesday	Wednesday	Thursday	Friday	Individual Totals

This week's Team total: __________

Wise Action Tool #7

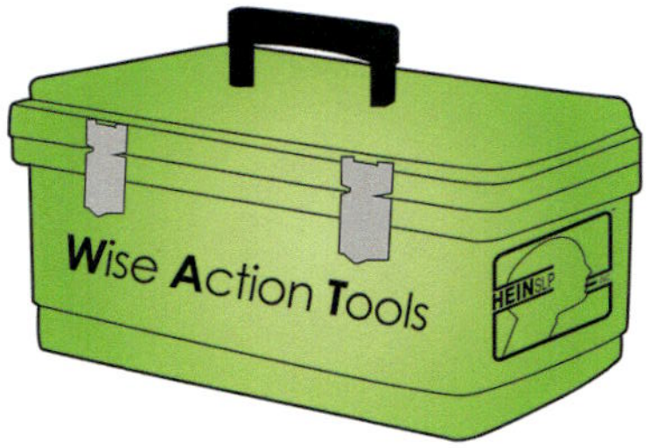

HOME TEAM G.R.E.E.N. ACTION TRACKER

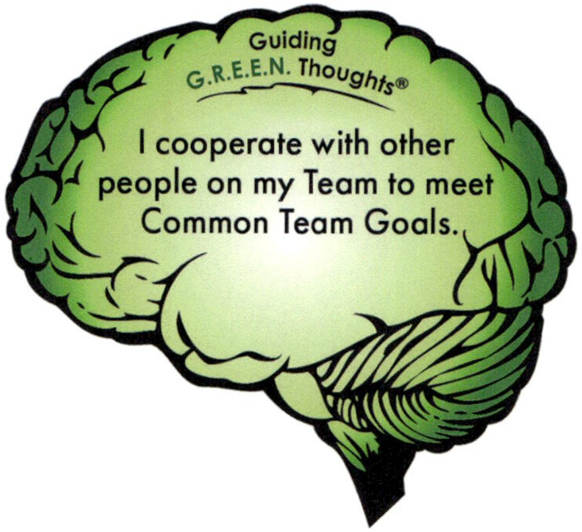

Name of our Home Team: ______________________________

This is our G.R.E.E.N. Action Tracker for the week starting on ______________
(date)

Fill in the names of all members of the Home Team. Fill out and then review the G.R.E.E.N. Action Reports. Put a check in a box to give a Home Team member credit on each date when he or she acted G.R.E.E.N.

Home Team Members	Mon	Tue	Wed	Thu	Fri	Sat	Sun	7-Day Total

This week's Home Team G.R.E.E.N. Action Total: ____________

Wise Action Tool #8

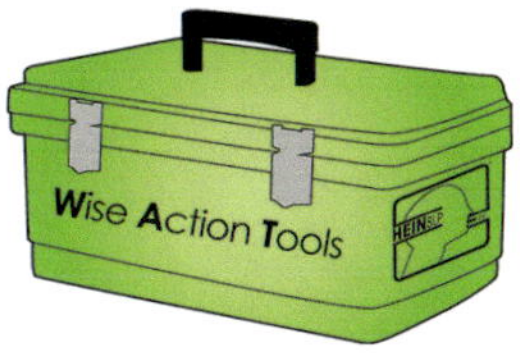

WORK TEAM G.R.E.E.N. ACTION TRACKER

Name of our Work Team: ______________________________

This is our Team Action Tracker for the week starting on ________________
(date)

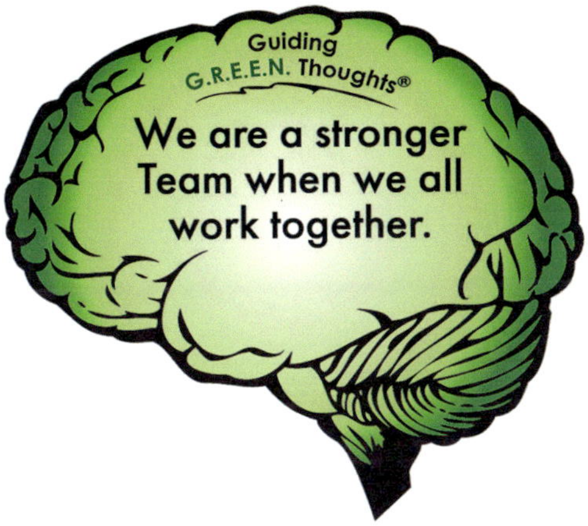

Fill in the names of everyone on the Team.

√ Check the box under the date each time a Work Team member acted G.R.E.E.N. or transfer the total from each Team member's Personal G.R.E.E.N. Action Tracker.

Work Teammates	Mon	Tue	Wed	Thu	Fri	Sat	Sun	Individual Totals

This week's Team total: ____________

Wise Action Tool #9

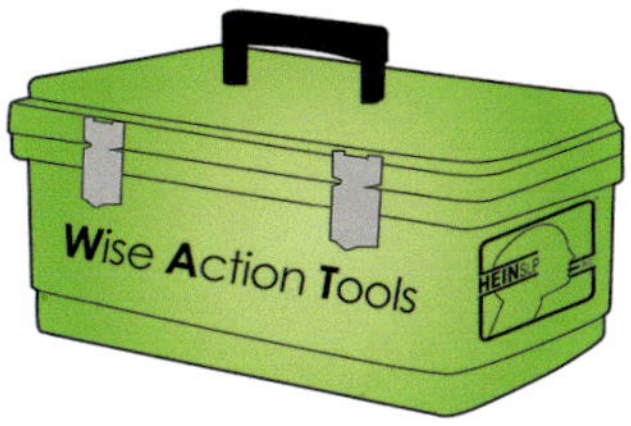

OUR CLASSROOM TEAM RULES

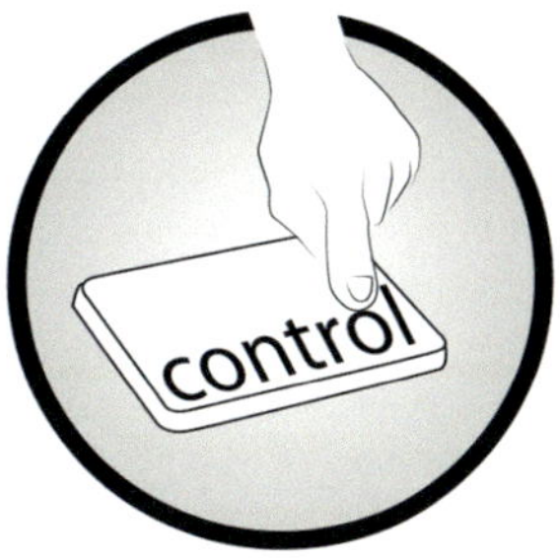

Everyone on our Classroom Team works to find the control to follow our Classroom Team rules.

These are the Classroom Team rules everyone on the Team follows so our Team can be great and powerful and keep moving forward!

1. ______________________________
   ____

2. ______________________________
   ____

3. ______________________________
   ____

4. ______________________________
   ____

5. ______________________________
   ____

Wise Action Tool #10

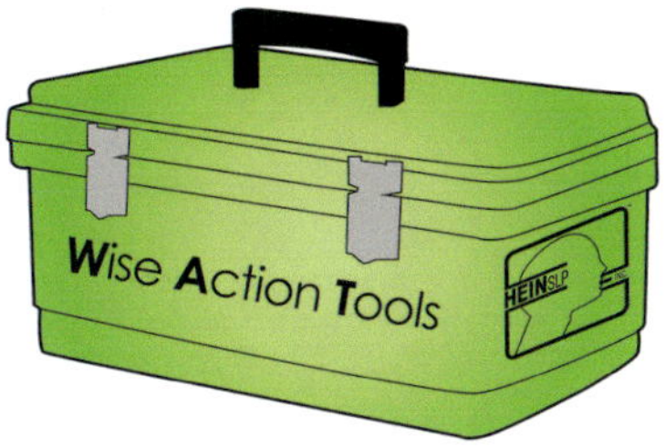

OUR HOME TEAM RULES

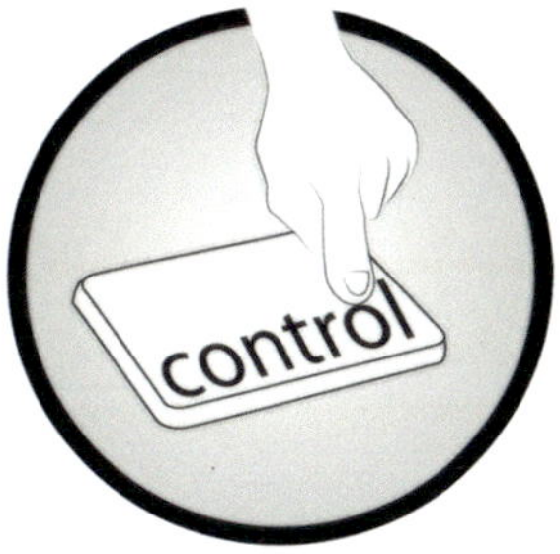

Everyone on our Home Team uses **self-control** and follows our Home Team Rules.

Here are our Home Team Rules.

Everyone on the Team follows these rules so our Team can be great and **powerful** and keep moving **forward**!

1. ______________________________

____

2. ______________________________

____

3. ______________________________

____

4. ______________________________

____

5. ______________________________

____

Wise Action Tool #11

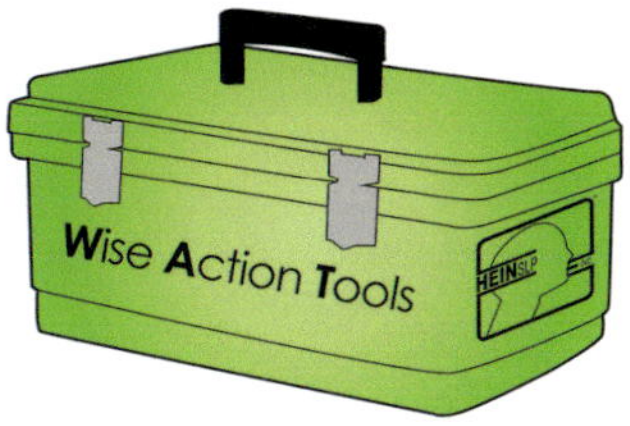

OUR FRIENDSHIP TEAM RULES

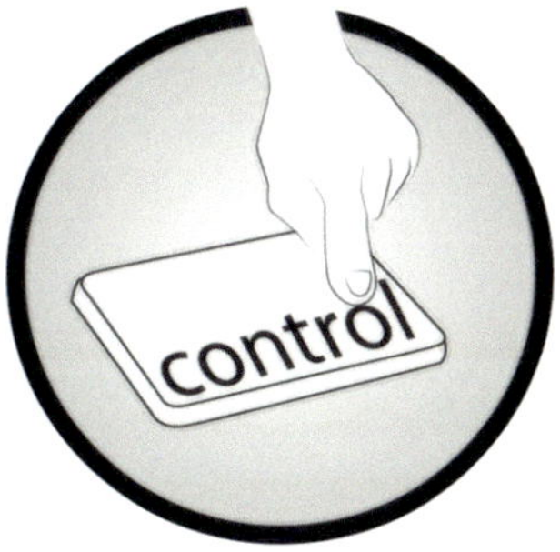

Everyone on our Friendship Team uses **self-control** and follows our Friendship Team Rules.

These are our Friendship Team Rules.

Everyone on the Team follows these rules so our Team can be great and **powerful** and keep moving **forward**!

1. ______________________________

____

2. ______________________________

____

3. ______________________________

____

4. ______________________________

____

5. ______________________________

____

Wise Action Tool #12

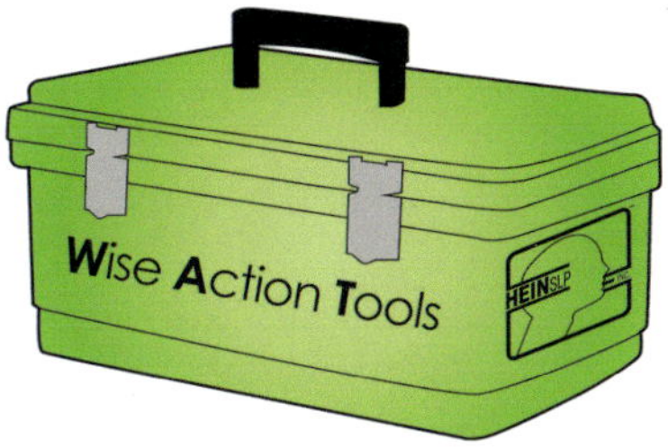

OU R WORK TEAM RULES

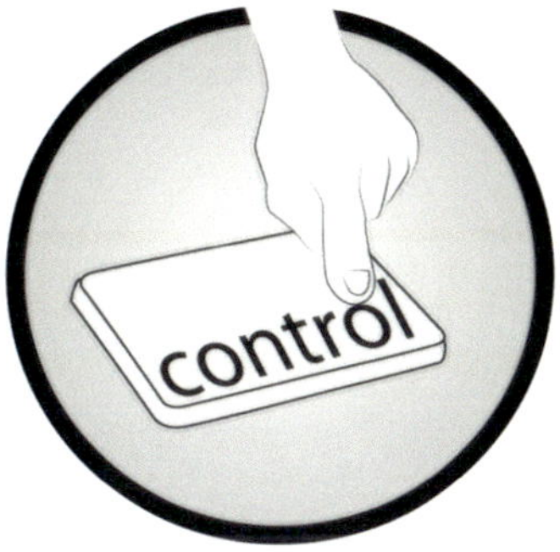

These are the Work Team Rules that everyone on our Team follows so our Team can be great and powerful and keep moving forward.

1. ____

____

2. ____

____

3. ____

____

4. ____

____

5. ____

____

Wise Action Tool #13

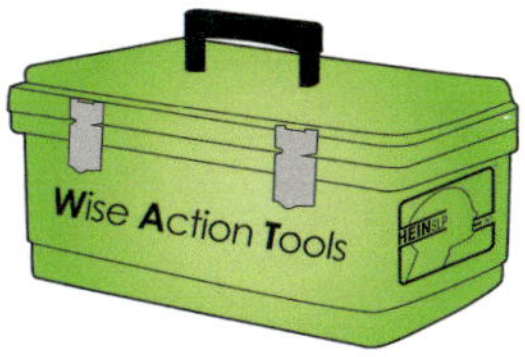

SELF-CHECK:
ARE YOU MAKING YOUR BEST LIFE STORY?

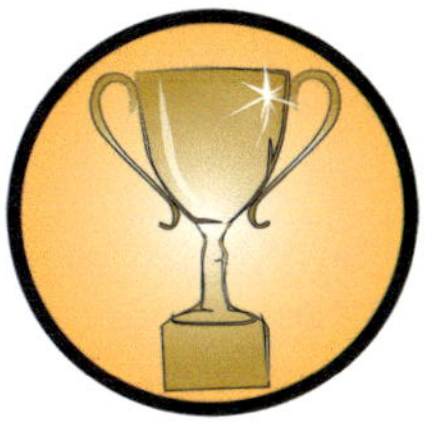

Answer these questions to help you think about whether you are making choices to help *your* life story be the best it can be:

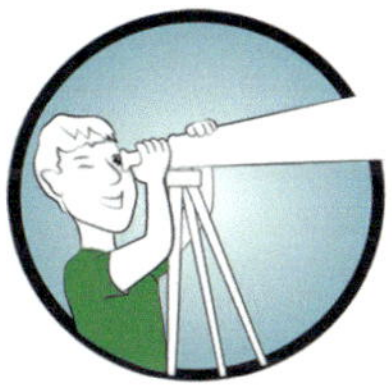

1. As the main character in your own life, are you alert and **paying attention to what's happening around you**?

   most of the time/ some of the time/ never

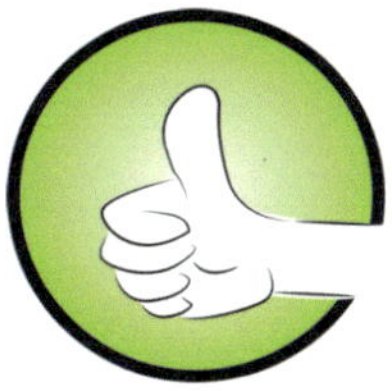

2. As the main character in your own life, are you making your best decisions so your life story gets **better**?

   most of the time/ some of the time/ never

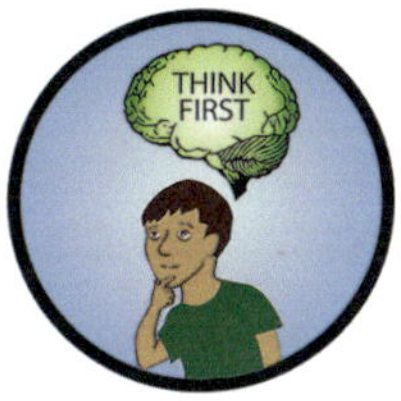

3. Do you think about acting **G.R.E.E.N.** in your own life story? Do you think about helping the other people in your life have **better** life stories too?

   most of the time/ some of the time/ never

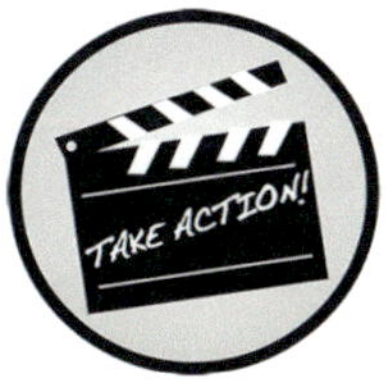

4. As the main character in your own life, do you take **positive** action when things need to be solved or fixed so each scene can be the best it can be?

   most of the time/ some of the time/ never

To be your **best self** in each scene in your own life story, you can follow these steps. The more you practice these skills, the more you strengthen the pathways in your brain that guide you to take **positive** action.

Wise Action Tool #14 (page 1)

IT IS NEVER TOO LATE TO START GUIDING YOURSELF TO BE THE BEST CHARACTER IN YOUR OWN BEST LIFE STORY!!! You have the **power** to choose the best action more often.

Think about making a **change** for the **better.** 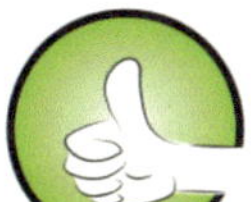 Every day you have the **power** to guide yourself to be the **best character** in your own **best life** story!!

Learn to make choices for your own **best life.** Act **G.R.E.E.N.** with others around you. It will change your attitude about what can happen each day. When you see **positive** things happening because of your actions, you will notice more **positive** energy growing inside of you. This will help you take the next steps toward the **best life** for yourself and people on your TEAMS.

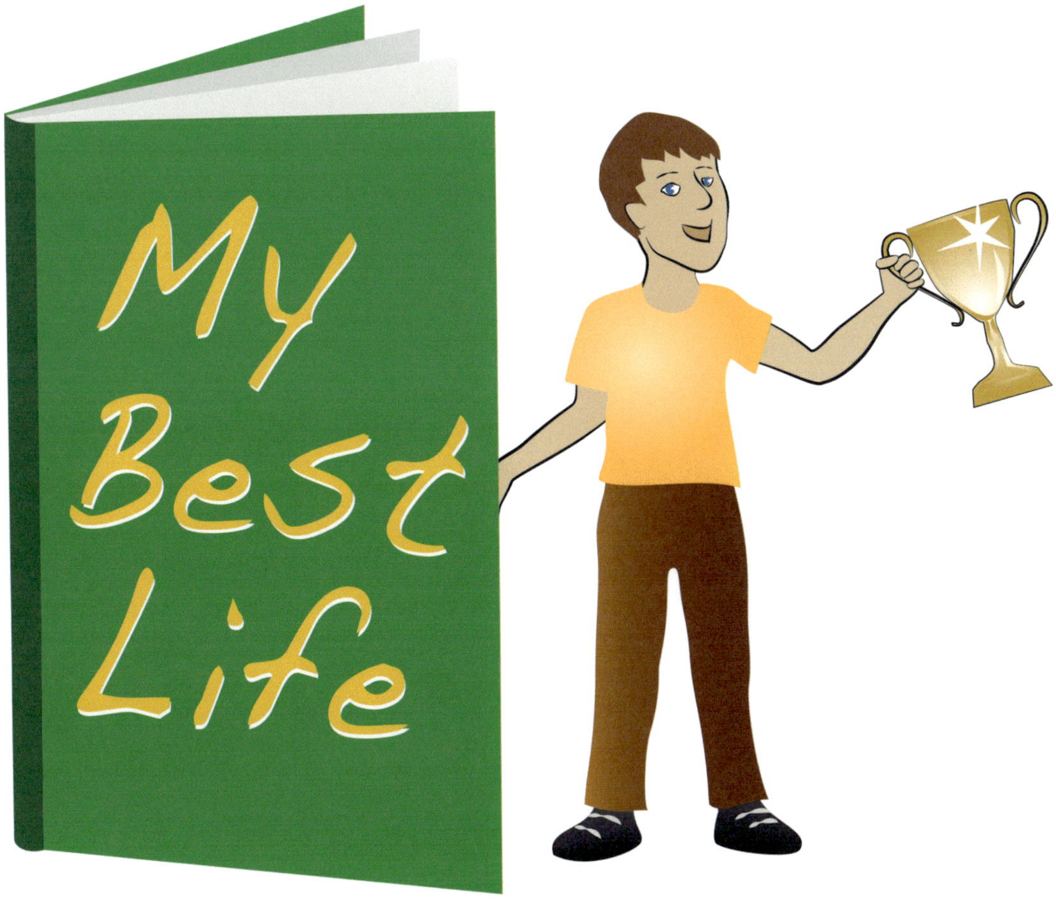

Wise Action Tool #14 (page 2)

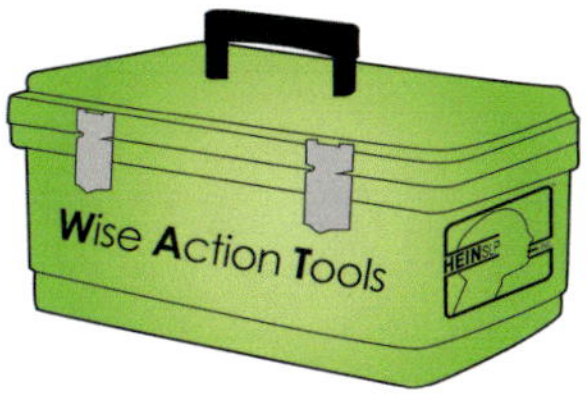

PICTURE YOUR OWN BEST LIFE!

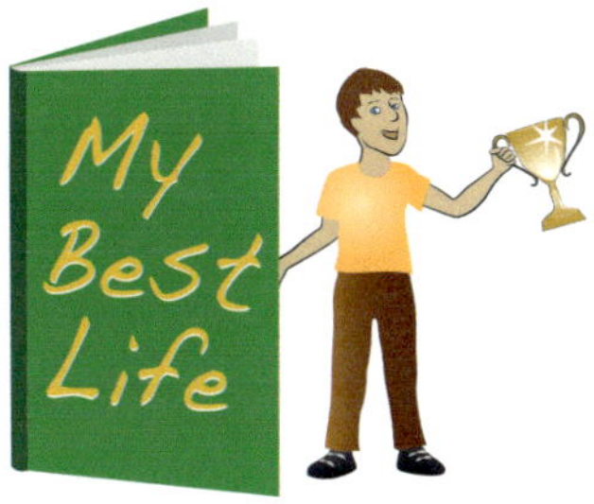

Now see if you can picture your own **best life**.

1. **Where** is your **best life** happening?
2. **Who** is with you in your own **best life**?
3. **What** are you doing in your life that makes it the best?
4. **When** is this **best life** of yours happening?

   tomorrow   next week   next month   next year   in five years

5. Draw your own **best life** in the box below or write in the words that describe the life you want to have. Start taking the road to your best life by taking your best steps in each and every one of your life scenes.

This is a picture of my own **best life**:

Wise Action Tool #15

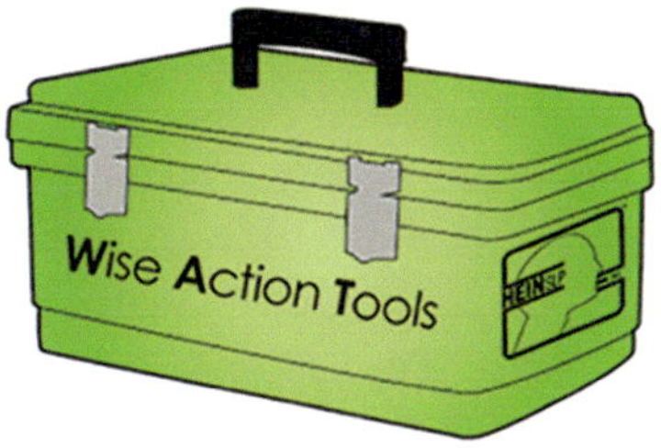

MY PERSONAL GOAL WORKSHEET

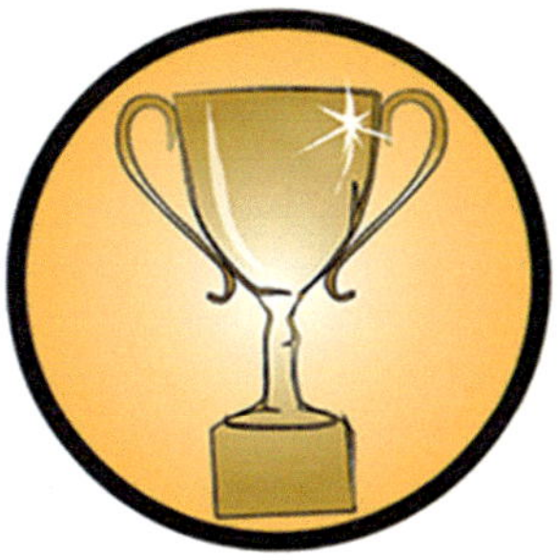

Today's Date: ______________________

Goal area: ____

My useful, realistic **goal** for the next week/month is: ____________________

____

A. Baseline: Circle how often I do it today.

Never sometimes half of the time most of the time almost always

0 5 10 15 20 25 30 35 40 45 **50** 55 60 65 70 75 80 85 90 95 **100**

B. My realistic **goal** for the next week/month is to do this ____________
(how often?)

Never sometimes half of the time most of the time almost always

My Goal: How often will I be able to do the action written in my goal
(circle how far you can *realistically* move to the right):

0 5 10 15 20 25 30 35 40 45 **50** 55 60 65 70 75 80 85 90 95 **100**

- -

Checking in: I am checking how I am doing on this date: ____________________

How am I doing? ____

What am I doing well? ____

What can help me do **better**? _____________________________________

Wise Action Tool #16

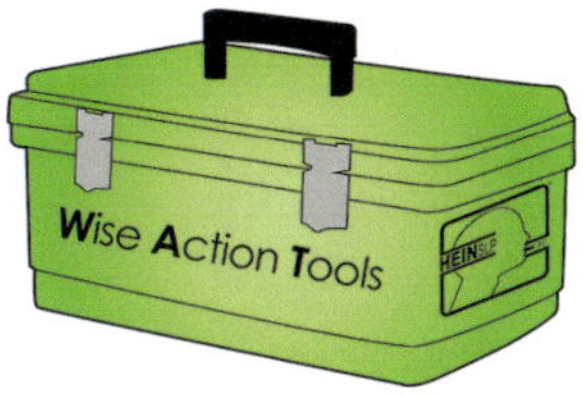

NOTING PROGRESS ON MY PERSONAL GOALS

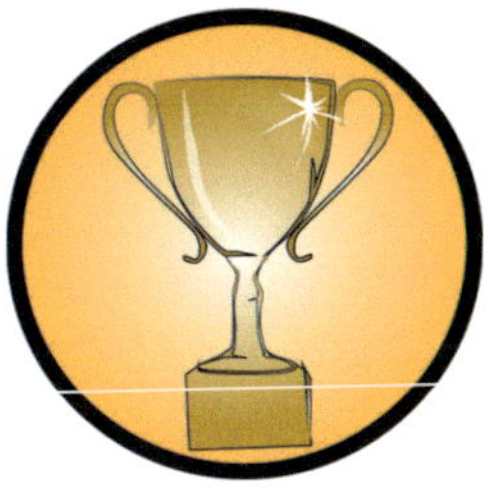

I am checking how I am doing on this date: ______________________________

How am I doing? What am I doing well? What can help me do better? __________

____

____

I am checking how I am doing on this date: ______________________________

How am I doing? What am I doing well? What can help me do better? __________

____

____

I am checking how I am doing on this date: ______________________________

How am I doing? What am I doing well? What can help me do better? __________

____

____

I am checking how I am doing on this date: ______________________________

How am I doing? What am I doing well? What can help me do better? __________

____

____

Wise Action Tool #17

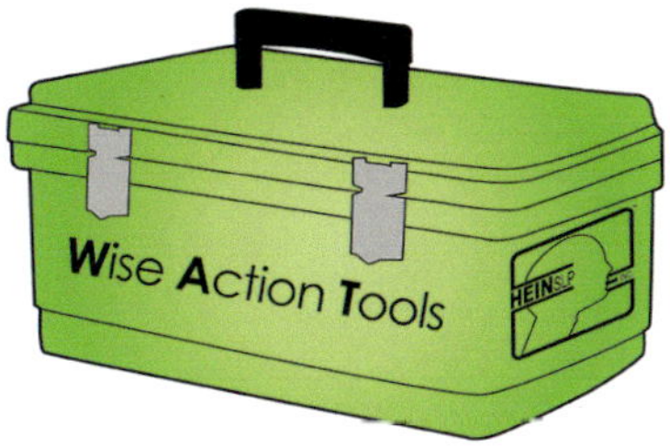

READY, SET, GOAL!

MY GOAL FOR RIGHT NOW

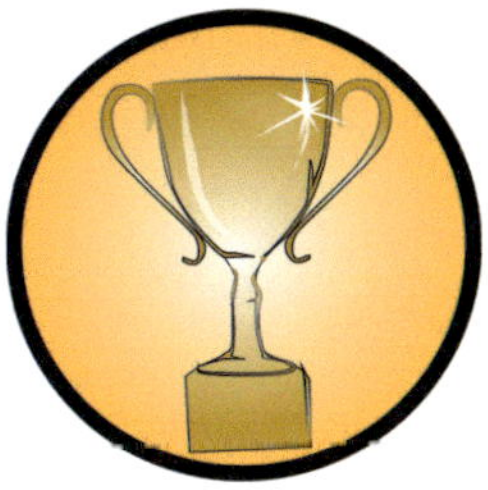

Name ______________________________ Date ____________________

1. The Team ____

2. Common Team Goal to meet now ____________________________________
____

3. My Personal Goal to meet right now _________________________________
____

4. Guiding G.R.E.E.N. Thought to help me meet my goal right now:

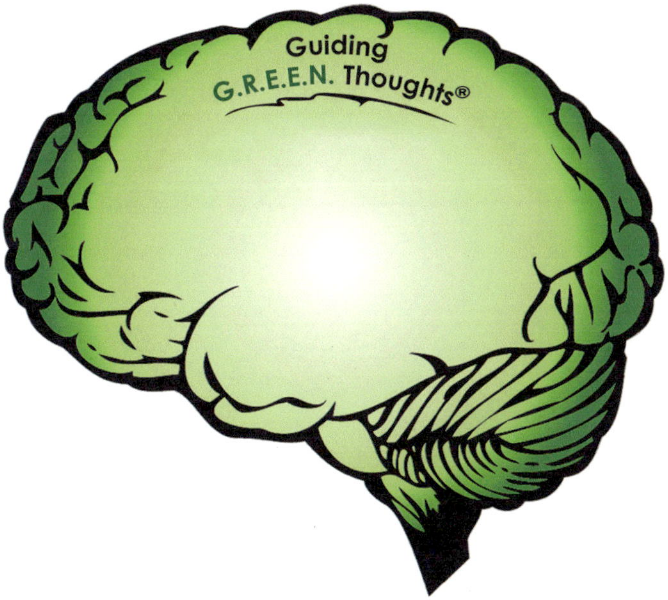

5. Take Action! 

6. How did I do? ____

   What did I do well? ____

   What could I do next time to be even more successful? ____________
   ____

Wise Action Tool #18

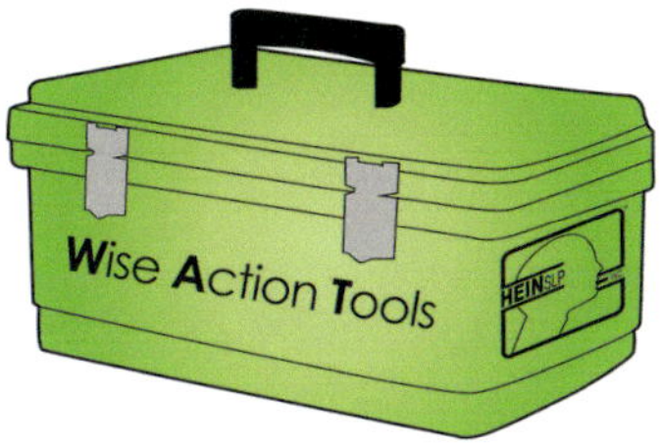

I DRAW MYSELF USING A GUIDING G.R.E.E.N. THOUGHT

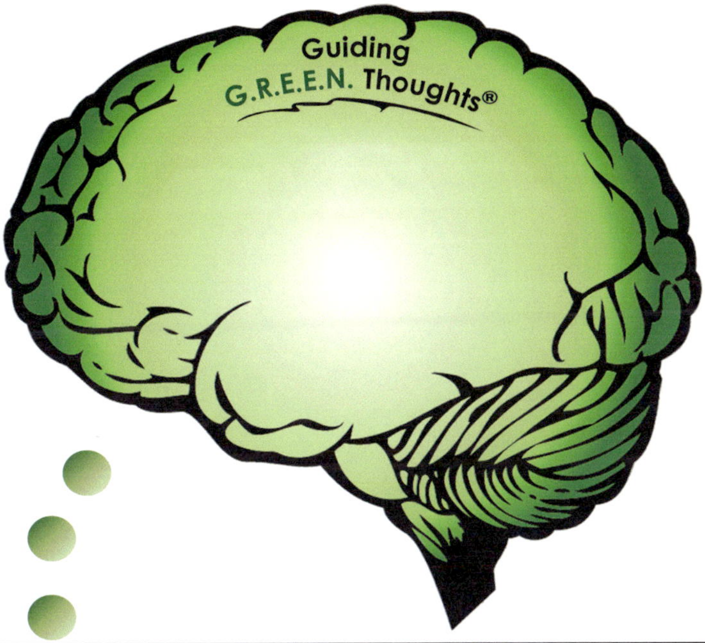

Here's a situation in which I am using a **Guiding G.R.E.E.N. Thought** so I can be the **best** I can be with my Team.

I am being my **better self** in a **better world**!

Wise Action Tool #19

GUIDING G.R.E.E.N. THOUGHT MEMORY CHALLENGE

Choose your most important **Guiding G.R.E.E.N. Thoughts®**. After reading them a few times, challenge yourself to write out what they are without looking at them. Write a "key" word from each thought that helps you picture the whole idea. Keep challenging yourself to remember all your important **Guiding G.R.E.E.N. Thoughts**. This will help you use them when needed.

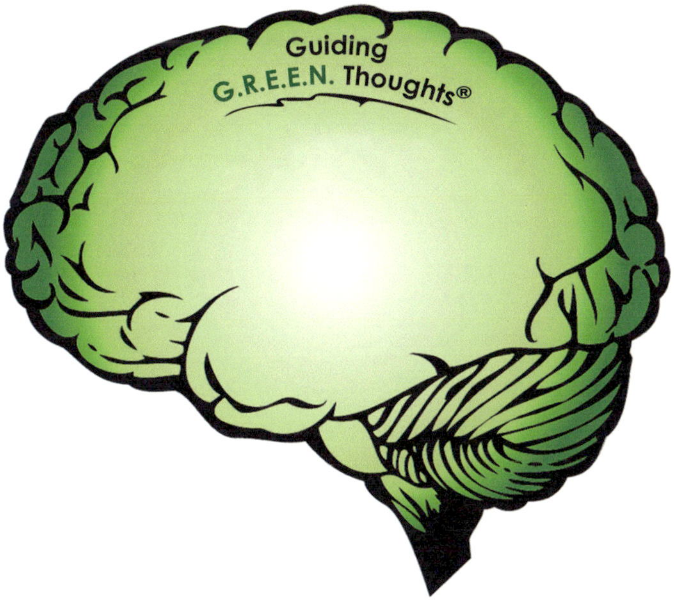

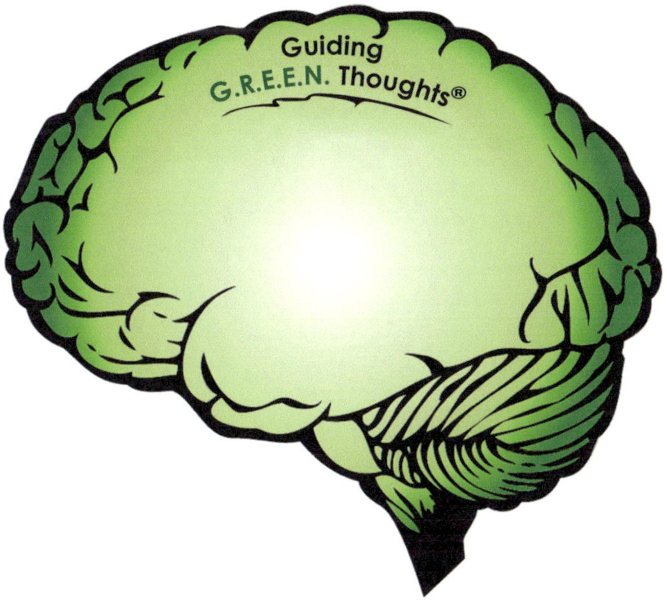

1. Key word ______________________

2. Key word ______________________

3. Key word ______________________

4. Key word ______________________

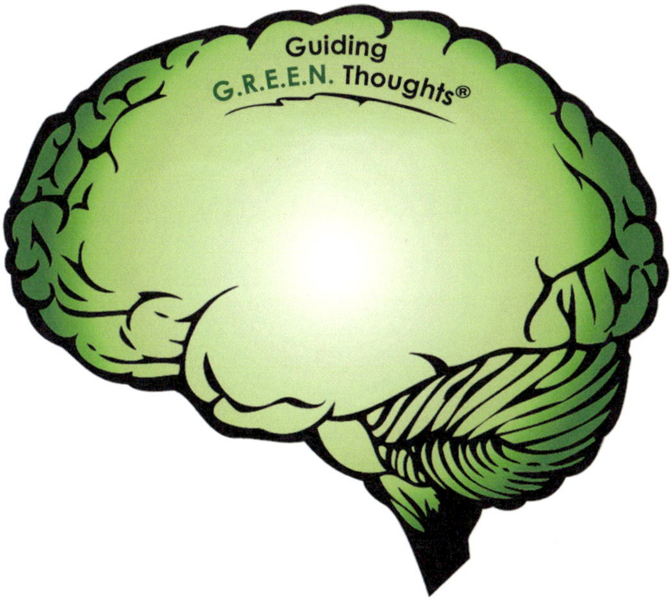

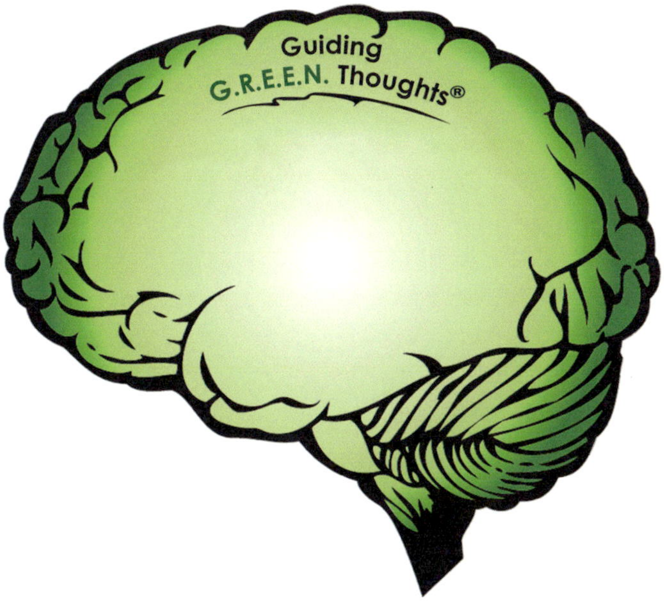

Wise Action Tool #20

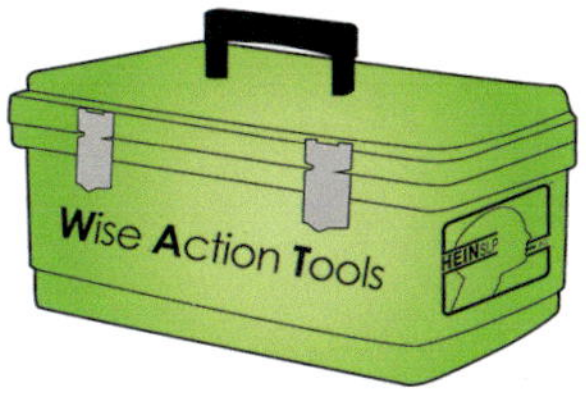

CIVILIZED CHOICE CHECKER

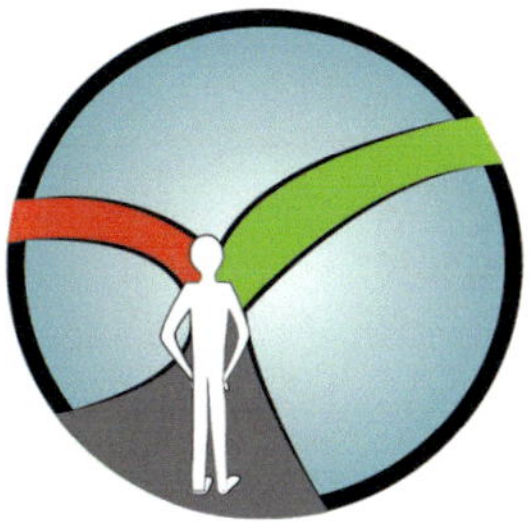

When I **survey this scene**, I think this is happening:

____

This is one way to act (**Choice A**): ______________________________

____

This is another way to act (**Choice B**): ____________________________

____

	Write "**+**" for **yes** and "**-**" for **no**	
	Action Choice A	Action Choice B
1. This is a logical choice. Things will get better instead of worse.		
2. This is a safe choice. People will *not* get hurt. Things will *not* get broken.		
3. This choice is **good for everyone**. Things will be better for *everyone* in the scene.		
4. This choice uses good **self-control** to meet the **goals**.		
Total score: Add up the **+** signs to see which choice is the best. Which choice wins?		

Wise Action Tool #21

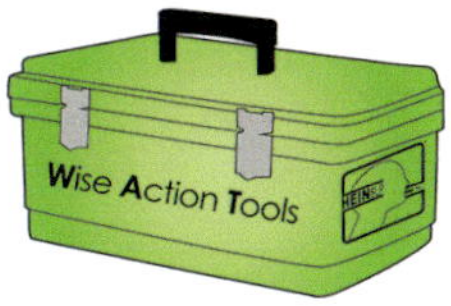

SURVEYING THE SCENE BEFORE TAKING ACTION

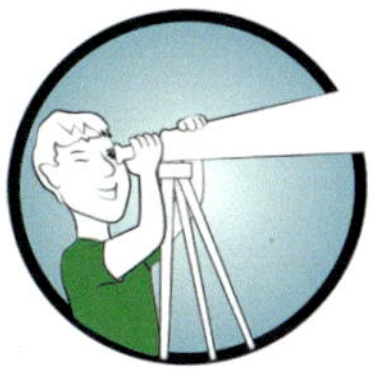

Directions: As you read each G.R.E.E.N. Scene, find clues to help you answer the following questions. This will help you know how to act in the scene.

1. The name of this G.R.E.E.N. Scene is ______________________________

2. What is the setting (where is this scene happening)? ______________________________

____

3. Who are the characters (who is in this scene)? ______________________________

____

4. What kind of Team is in this scene? Home Team School Team Friendship Team

5. What does each character in this scene want or need? ______________________________

____

____

____

6. What do you think is the Common Team Goal in this scene? ______________________________

____

7. What would be a positive consequence of everyone in the scene doing their best to act G.R.E.E.N.?

____

____

Wise Action Tool #22

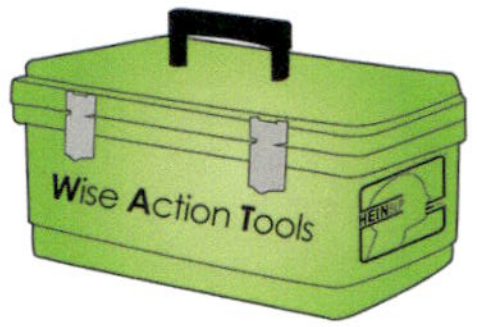

G.R.E.E.N. SCENE REVIEW FORM

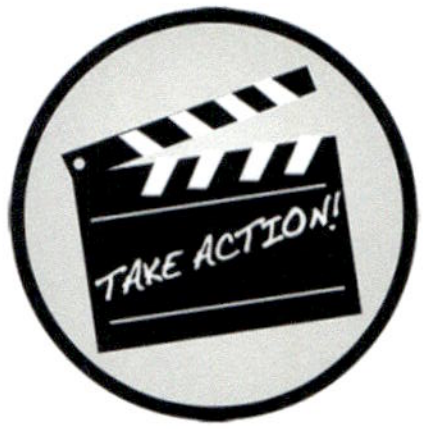

Date ____________________ Name of Reviewer ____________________

Name of G.R.E.E.N. Scene/Situation ____________________

The goal of this "Team" ____________________

G.R.E.E.N. SCENE TEAM MEMBER	ROLE IN THIS SCENE	G Grateful said "thank you" or otherwise showed appreciation	R Respectful used polite words and tone of voice	E Empathetic acted as if they cared about the other people	E Easygoing acted cooperatively to help achieve the TEAM goal	N Navigating stayed calm and handled a challenging situation
1.						
2.						
3.						

Comments—extra "takes" or cues needed? ____________________

Wise Action Tool #23

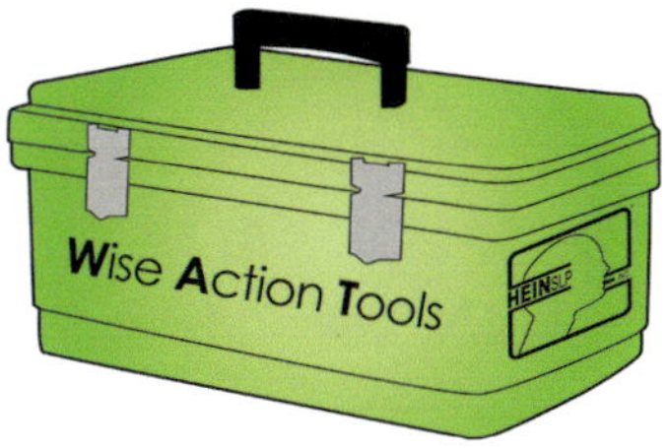

BRAKE TO TAKE A 5 BREAK

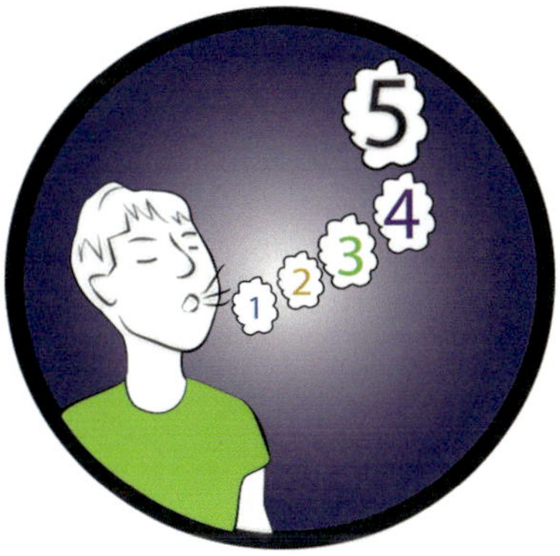

These are the steps for Braking to Take a 5 Break:

1. First, tell yourself to step on the brakes 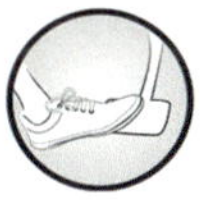 so you can avoid heading in the wrong direction. This will give you time to flip the switch 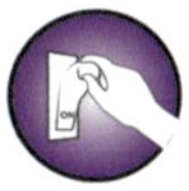 and change your direction.

2. Next, stop what you are doing so you can get ready to Take a 5 Break.

   Let your brain give your body a red light signal to avoid doing something without thinking. When you have stopped, you can remind yourself of your goals. When you become calm, you will survey the scene and move forward in the direction best for yourself and those around you.

3. You are ready for a 5 break.

   Concentrate on taking 5 controlled breaths. This is a powerful way to become calm. The only important thing for a few seconds is your breathing. You calm yourself by focusing all your attention on your breathing. You breathe in and out slowly 5 times. Start with at least 5 controlled breaths and repeat if you need to.

I breathe in slowly through my nose like just like I am breathing in the smell of fragrant flowers.

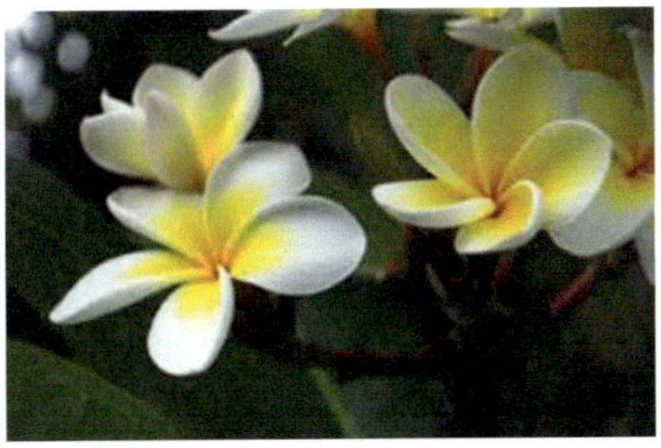

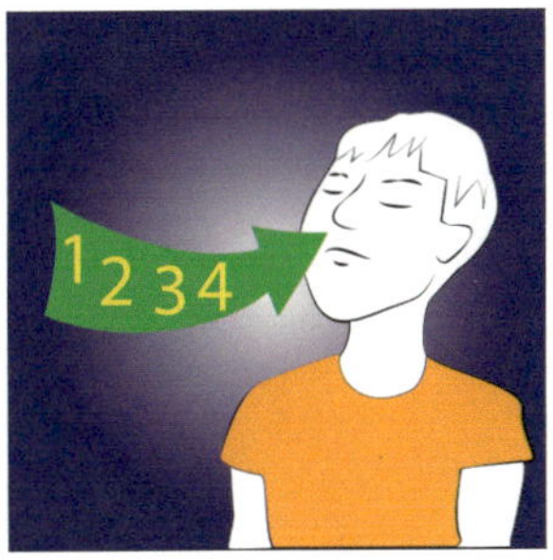

I count slowly to four: 1 . . . 2 . . . 3 . . . 4

Wise Action Tool #24 (page 1)

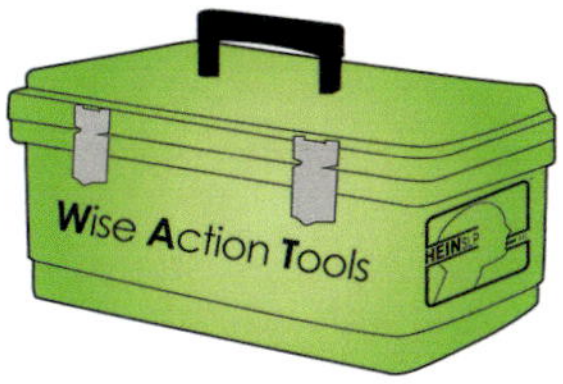

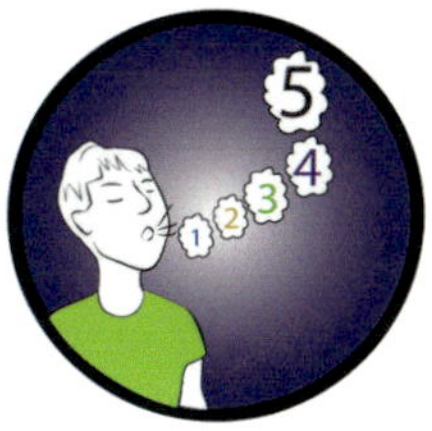

Then I breathe out slowly through my mouth as if I am blowing out many birthday candles.

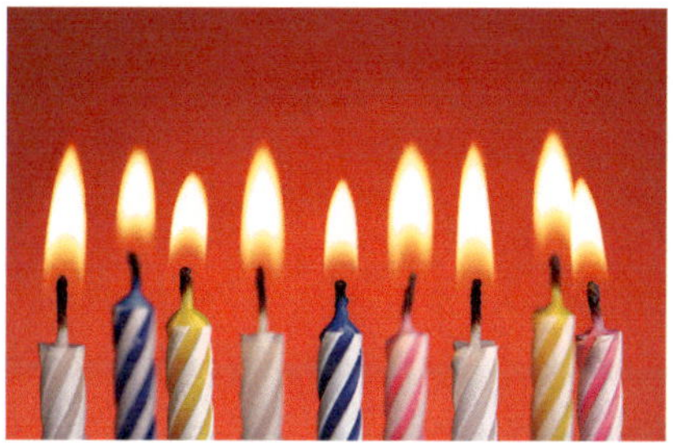

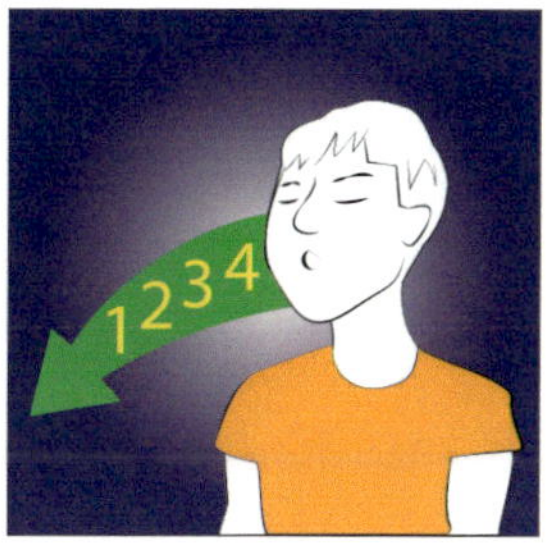

I count slowly to four: 1 . . . 2 . . . 3 . . . 4

4. When you listen to the "Brake to Take a 5 Break" song, it will help you do your controlled breathing with a calming rhythm. Each time you do this, you will get better at concentrating on the slow rhythm so it helps you get calmer:

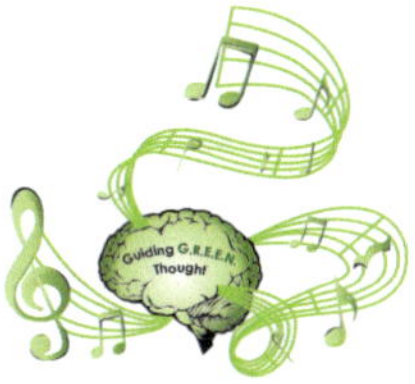

1. BREATHE in . . . 2 . . . 3 . . . 4 BREATHE out . . . 2 . . . 3 . . . 4

2. BREATHE in . . . 2 . . . 3 . . . 4 BREATHE out . . . 2 . . . 3 . . . 4

3. BREATHE in . . . 2 . . . 3 . . . 4 BREATHE out . . . 2 . . . 3 . . . 4

4. BREATHE in . . . 2 . . . 3 . . . 4 BREATHE out . . . 2 . . . 3 . . . 4

5. BREATHE in . . . 2 . . . 3 . . . 4 BREATHE out . . . 2 . . . 3 . . . 4

5. While doing your controlled breathing, you may do some other things with your body to help you get even more calm:

a. Count on your fingers while taking each of the five full breaths.

OR

b. Give yourself a full body hug while taking the five full breaths.

OR

c. Press your hands together while taking the five full breaths.

(Try each self-calming body movement to see which one helps you calm down the most.)

6. Once you feel calmer, you will be able to reach for **Guiding G.R.E.E.N. Thoughts** to successfully navigate the scene.

Wise Action Tool #24 (page 2)

PEACEFUL SCENES TO HELP ME STAY CALM

I feel more calm when I look at these pictures. I can think of these pictures at any time and any place when I want to self-calm and stay calm.

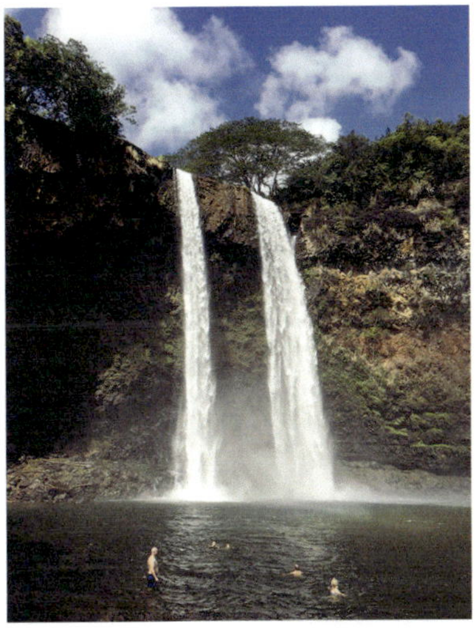

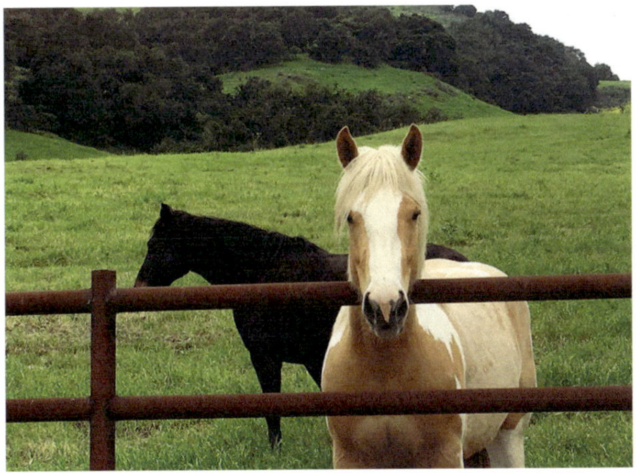

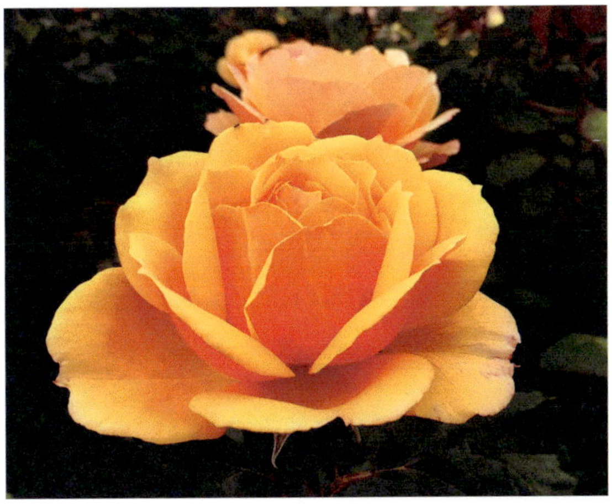

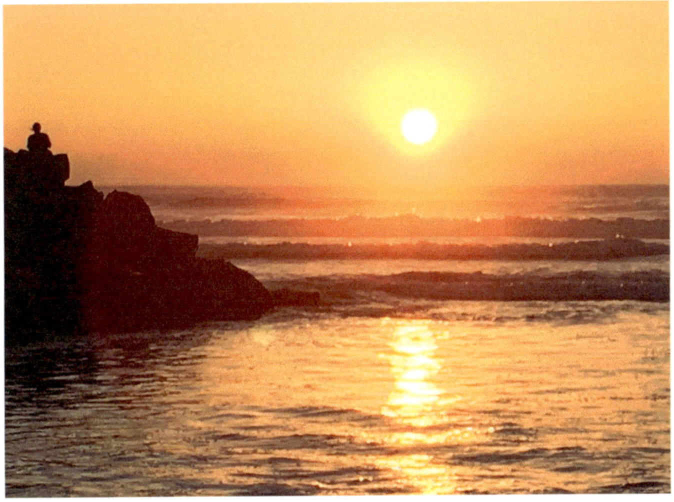

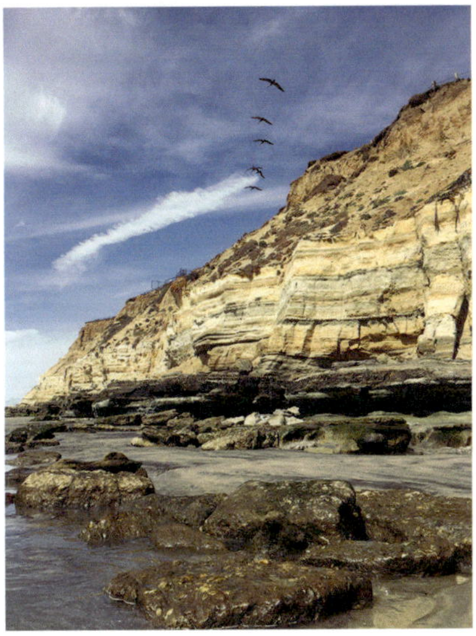

Wise Action Tool #25

CREATING MY OWN SELF-CALMING SCENE

This is a picture I have found or a drawing I have made that helps me feel calm (I can imagine taking a trip here whenever I need to, so I can get calm and stay calm).

Wise Action Tool #26

Wise Action Tools

THIS IS HOW I LOOK AFTER I USE A SELF-CALMING STRATEGY

This is a picture of me successfully being with my team *after* I use my self-calming strategy.

Wise Action Tool #27

SELF-CALMING BY QUIETLY SQUEEZING A FIDGET

If you are feeling hyper, and have a lot of extra energy, you can quietly squeeze a calming fidget tool in one of your hands to release some of your energy. This will help you get out some energy in a way that does not bother other people on your Team.

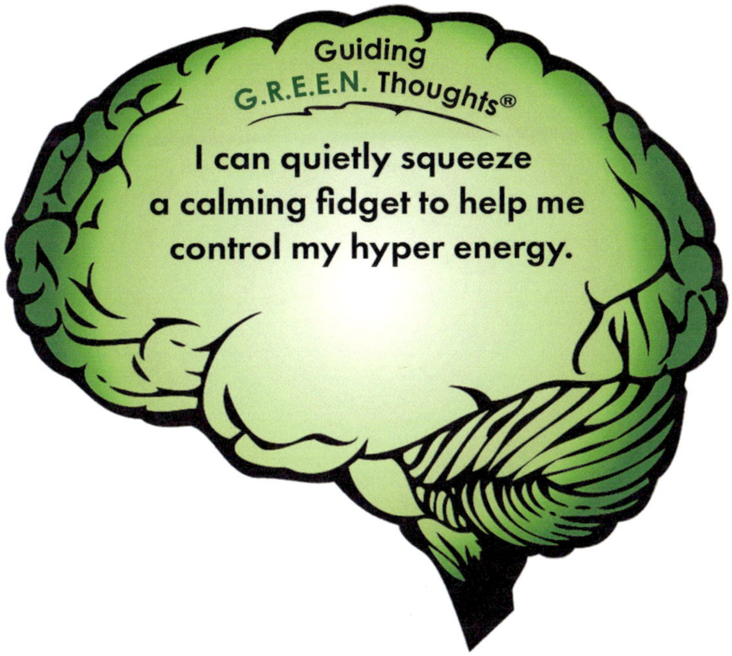

It takes practice to use a calming fidget tool quietly. It is easy to forget to get your body calmer and *not* to get acting *more* hyper! Quietly squeezing the fidget can calm your body to help you focus. But, you have to learn self-control so you don't bounce it, or throw it, or drop it and distract yourself and other people on your Team.

Practice using the fidget tool in the right way with your **powerful self-control**, so it can help you focus!

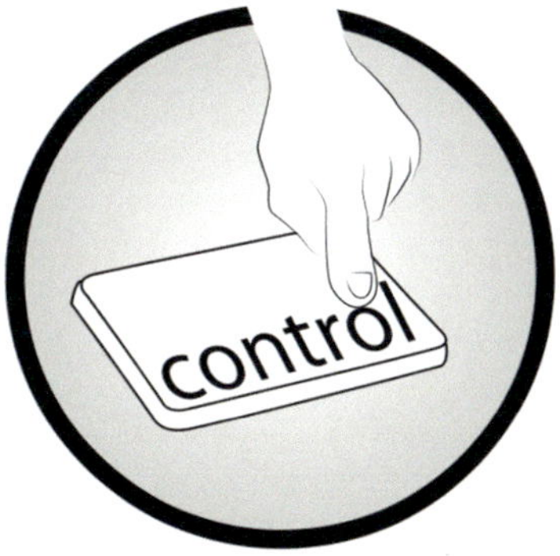

Wise Action Tool #28

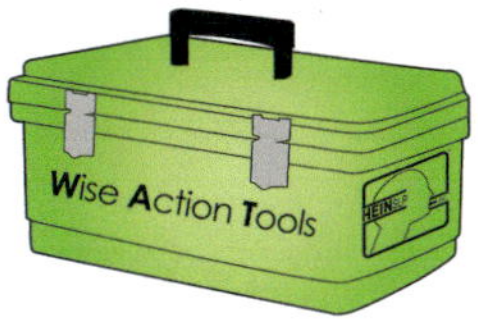

WRITING YOUR OWN GUIDING G.R.E.E.N. THOUGHT FOR SELF-CONTROL

You can write your own **Guiding G.R.E.E.N. Thought** that can help you control your body.

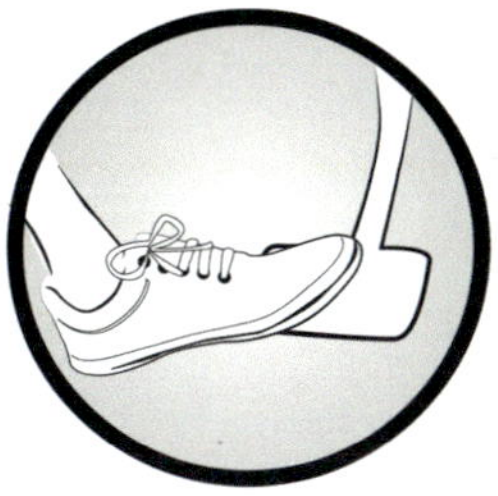

If you are making noises, saying words, or acting in ways that are bothering someone else, you can **step on the brakes** and use a **Wise Action Tool** instead. You can find a **Guiding G.R.E.E.N. Thought** and take your best action. Sometimes you will find that your best action is to stop an action!

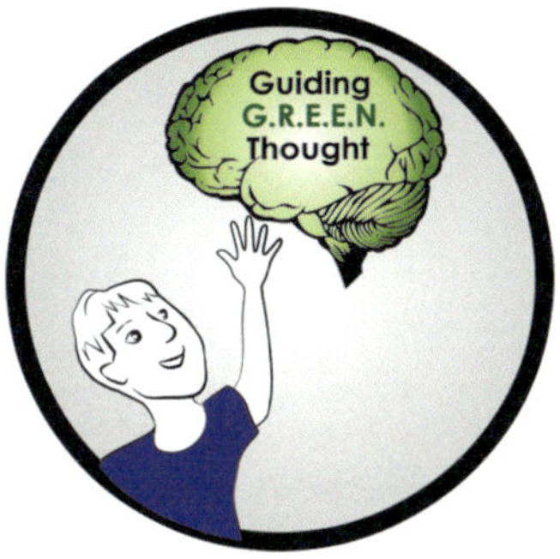

You can also write your own thought and tell why your **Guiding G.R.E.E.N. Thought** will help you and your Team. The most important step will be to actually do what the **Guiding G.R.E.E.N. Thought** says!

The more you practice controlling your body to stop action that is bothering other people, the more you realize that it really makes your scene **better**.

And the more you practice stopping any of your body's **negative** actions, the easier it will be to use **self-control** the next time you need it.

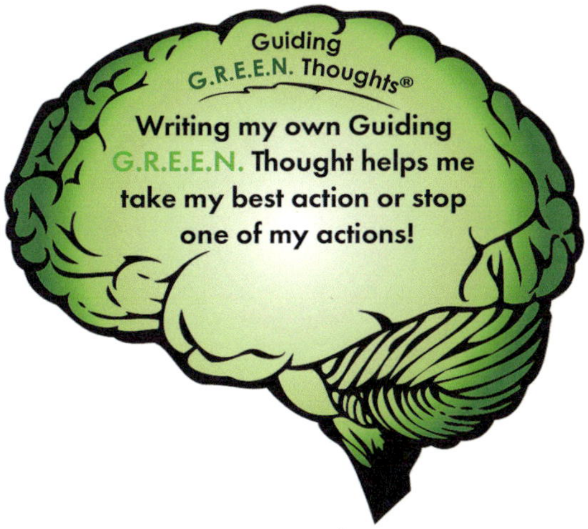

Wise Action Tool #29 (page 1)

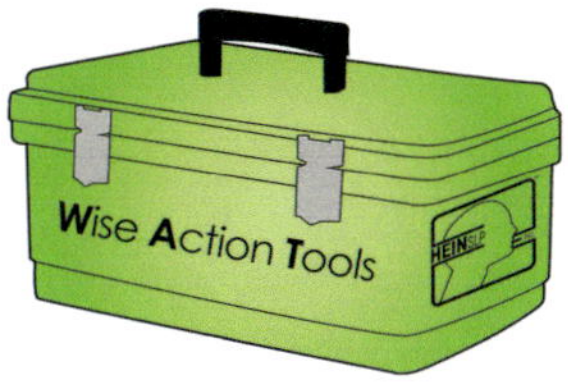

You can also write down your own thought and tell why your **Guiding G.R.E.E.N. Thought** will help you and your TEAM. The most important step will be to actually do what the **Guiding G.R.E.E.N. Thought** says!

The more you practice controlling your body to stop action that is bothering other people, the more you will realize that it really makes your scene **better**.

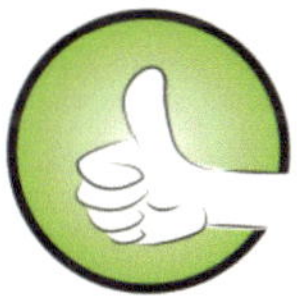

And the more you practice with your body, the easier it will be to use **self-control** the next time you need it.

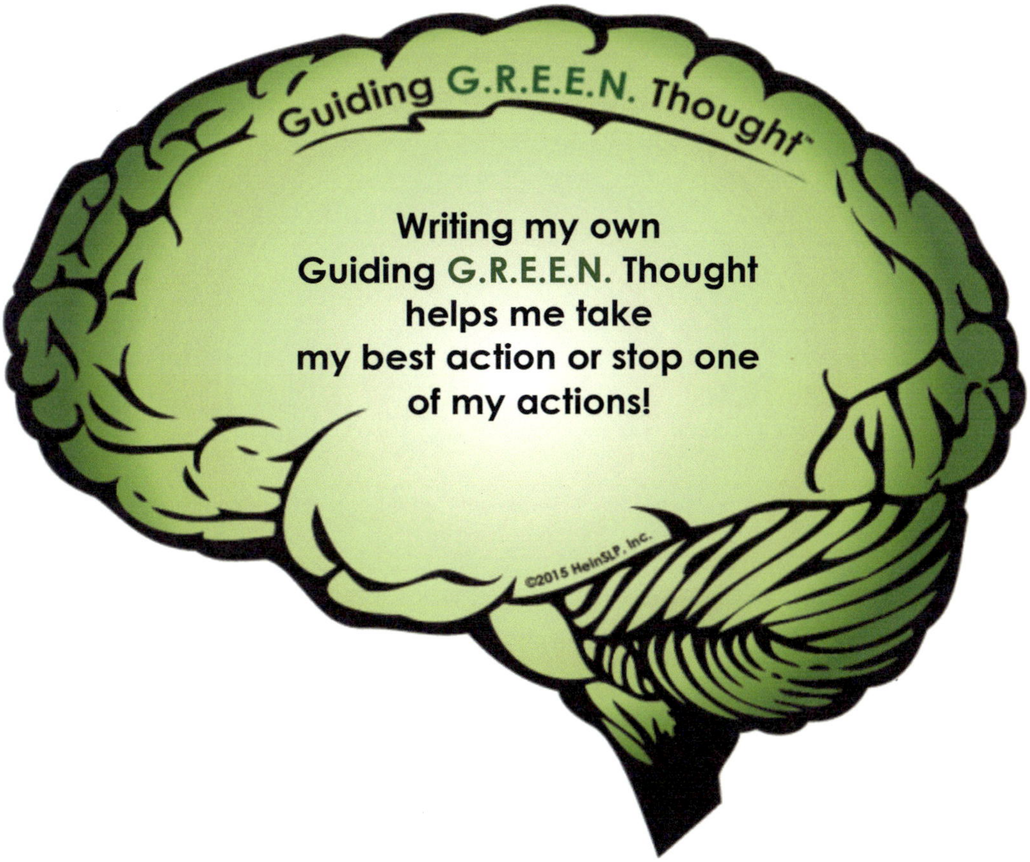

Wise Action Tool #29 (page 2)

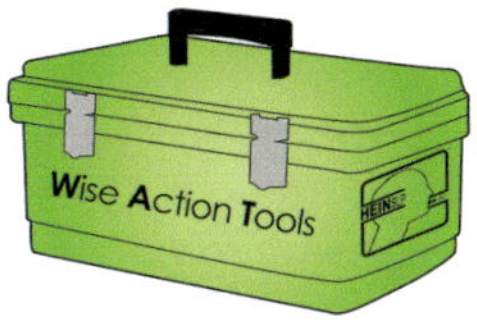

MY OWN GUIDING G.R.E.E.N. THOUGHT FOR HAVING SELF-CONTROL TO STOP HARMFUL ACTION

Here is my **Guiding G.R.E.E.N. Thought** to help me step on the brakes to stop any harmful actions I might be taking.

I have self-control to stop taking harmful actions so I can help my Team.

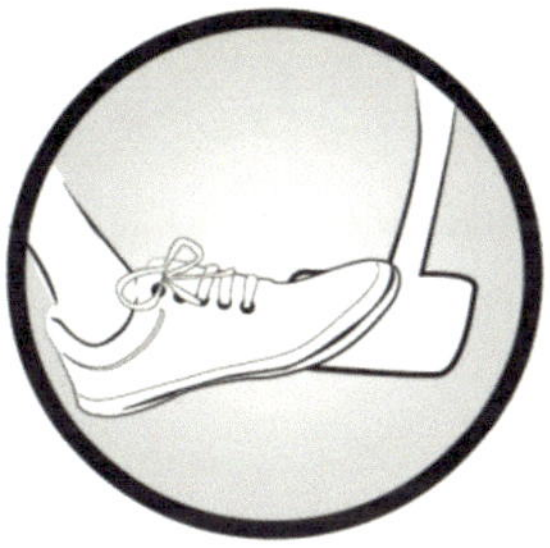

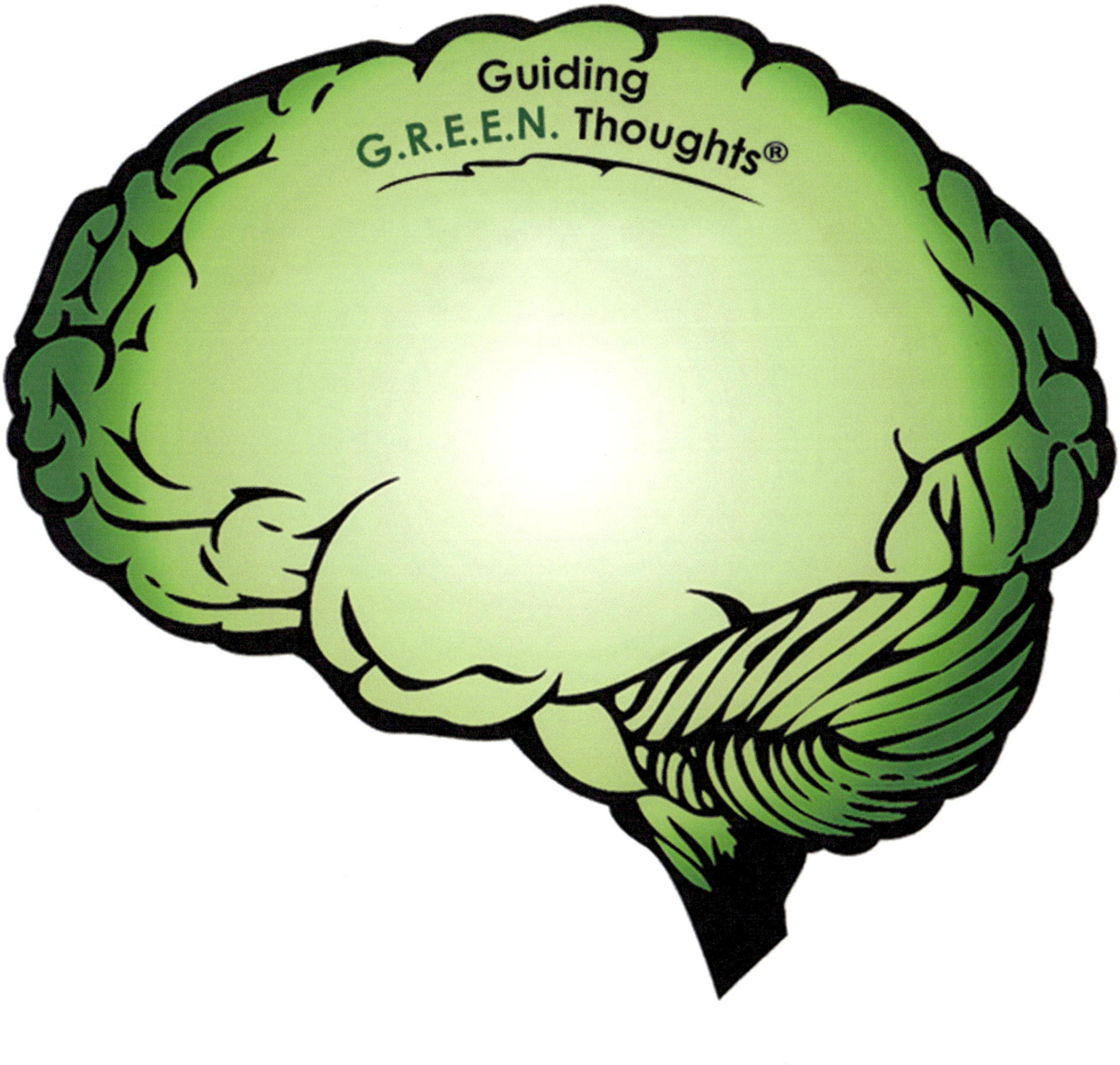

Wise Action Tool #30

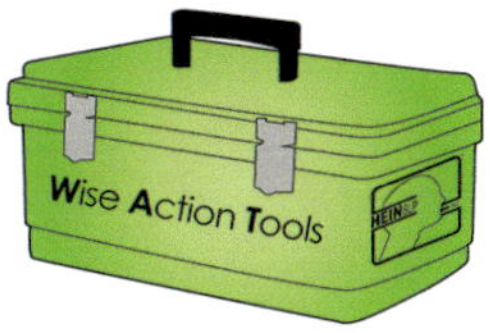

THOUGHT TRANSFORMATION SCENE CHANGER

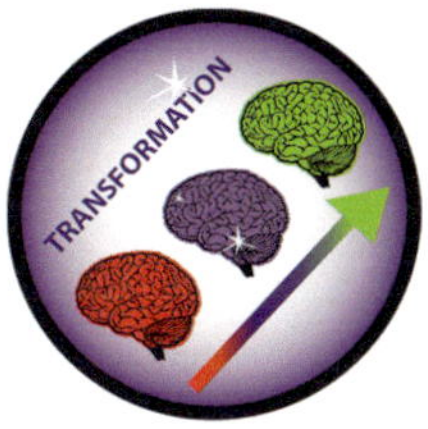

Name ______________________________ Date ____________________

1. The Scene at first, *before* G.R.E.E.N. Thought Transformation.

a. Write or draw how I am acting with other people in this scene *before* the **G.R.E.E.N.** Thought **Transformation**.

b. What feedback am I getting from others about my actions? ____________________

____

c. How are all the people in this scene feeling, including me? ____________________

____

2. Get the Power!

Change the scene!

Be **open-minded** to make a **Transformation**.

Think of Guiding **G.R.E.E.N.** Thoughts to make it happen!

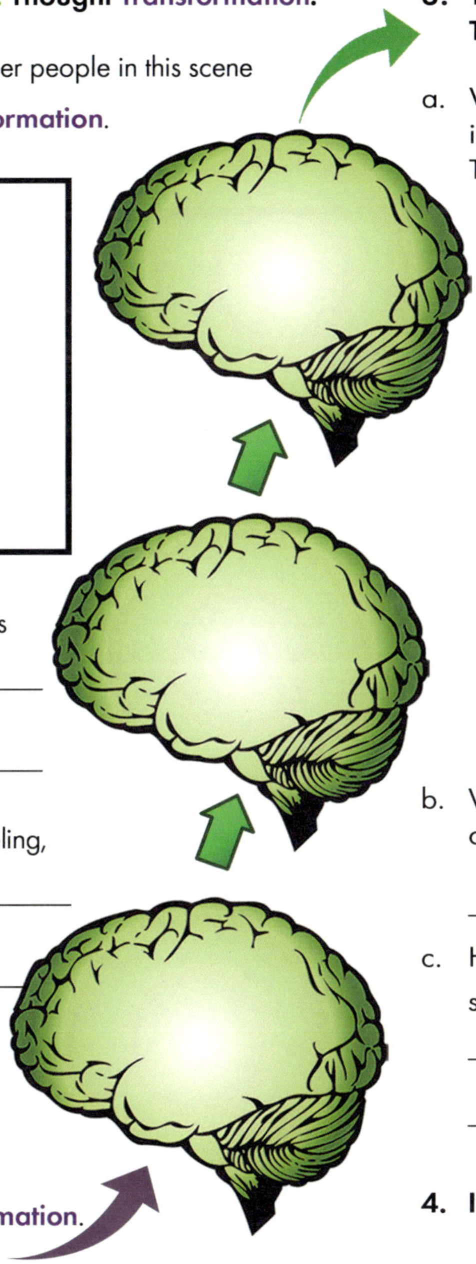

3. The new scene *after* G.R.E.E.N. Thought Transformation.

a. Write or draw what is happening in this scene *after* **G.R.E.E.N.** Thought **Transformation**.

b. What feedback am I getting from others about my actions? ____________________

____

c. How are all the people in this scene feeling now, including me?

____

____

4. Is this new scene better?

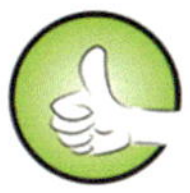

yes **no**

Why? ____________________

____

5. This page shows a powerful Transformation from ____________________ to ____________________.

Wise Action Tool #31

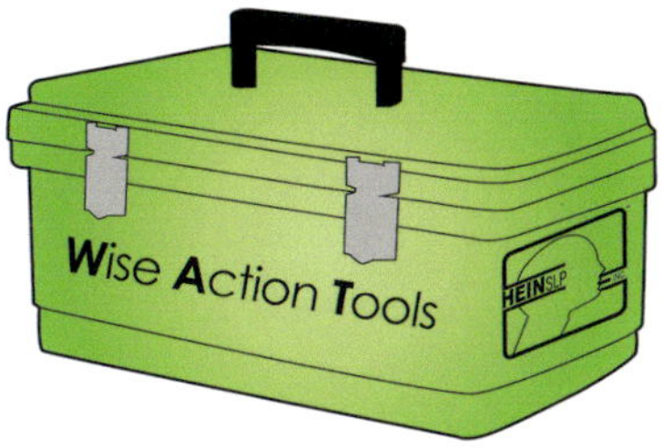

APPRECIATION BOX

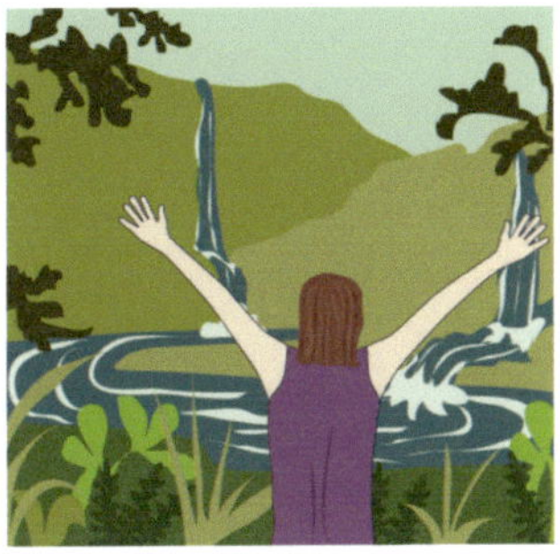

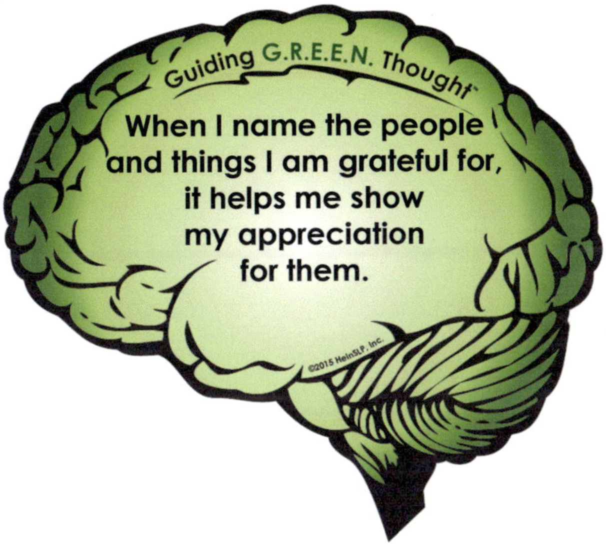

MY APPRECIATION BOX

This is a picture of me with the people and things that I am **grateful** for having in my life. I fill this box with everyone and everything I **appreciate**.
I am in this scene too, because I **appreciate** being alive!

Wise Action Tool #32

PLEASE TELL ME SOMETHING RIGHT AWAY WHEN I ASK YOU A QUESTION!

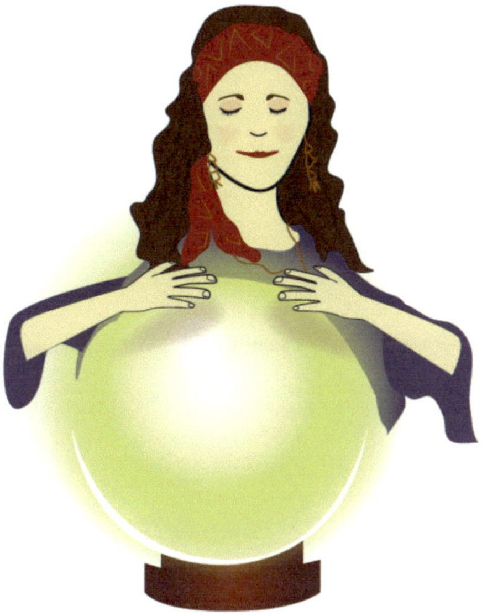

"Let me look into my crystal ball...
I try really hard, but I cannot read your mind."

Help me help you. Please do one of the following after I ask you a question:

1. Quickly tell me the answer if you know it. **The answer is . . .**

or

2. Say, **"Wait a minute, please. I'm thinking"** if you need more time to think.

or

3. Say, **"Please tell me again"** if you did not hear what I said.

or

4. Say, **"I don't know. I need some help answering the question"** if you don't know how to answer the question correctly.

Wise Action Tool #33

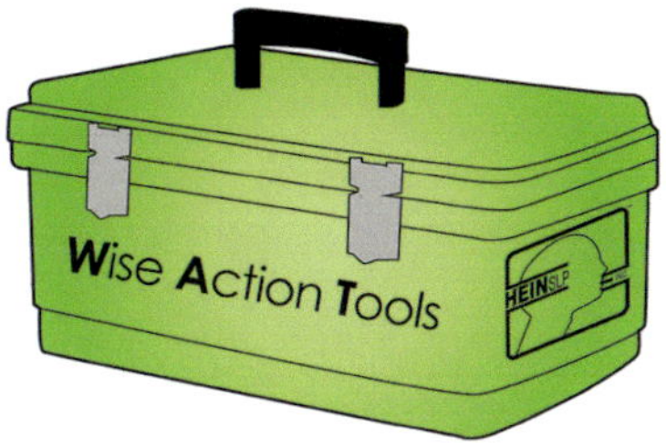

ON-TOPIC TRACKER

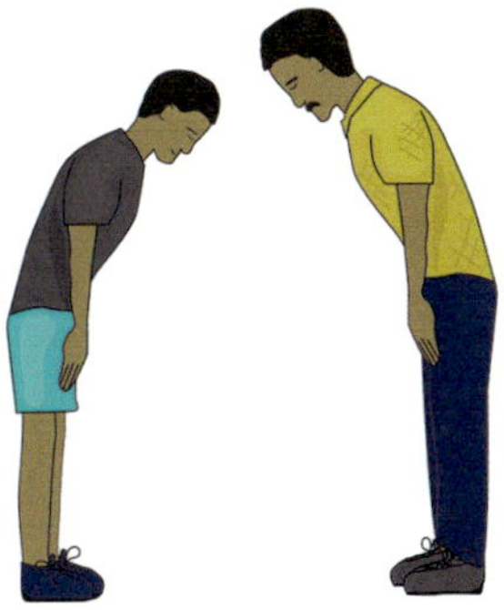

1. What is this Conversation **Team** Topic? ______________________________

____

2. Fill in the names of the conversation partners and check when each partner asks a question or makes a comment that relates to the **Team** topic. Check on the bottom if each partner stayed **on-topic** or went off-topic during this conversation.

____________ CONVERSATION PARTNER #1	____________ CONVERSATION PARTNER #2
____ question(s) asked about the Team topic __ __ __ __ __	____ question(s) asked about the Team topic __ __ __ __ __
____ comments made about the Team topic __ __ __ __ __	____ comments made about the Team topic __ __ __ __ __
ON-TOPIC OFF-TOPIC	ON-TOPIC OFF-TOPIC

3. Did both conversation partners stay **on-topic**? yes no

4. After both conversation partners have stayed **on-topic** about one topic, they can start to have another **on-topic** conversation about a different topic.

Wise Action Tool #34

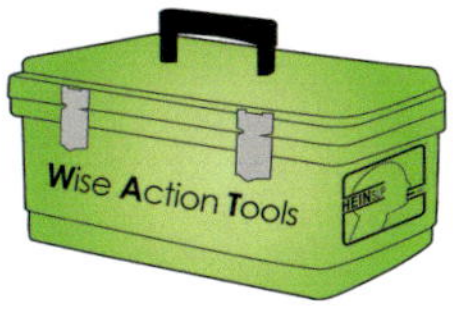

TAKE THE CONVERSATION POWER CHALLENGE!

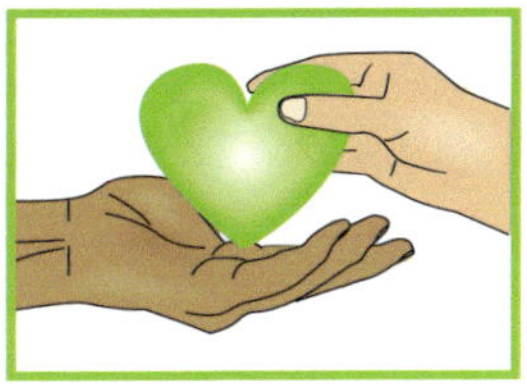

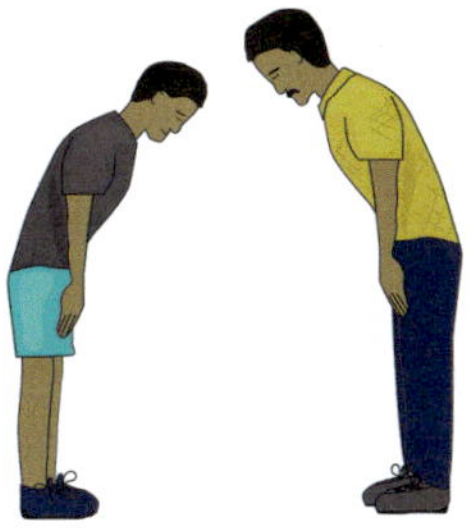

1. **TALK ABOUT A TOPIC THAT YOUR CONVERSATION PARTNER LIKES TO TALK ABOUT**—Challenge yourself to show that you **care** enough about someone else on one of your Teams by having a conversation with that person about a topic that is important to them. It may be a challenge for you because that topic may be one that has nothing to do with your own activities or interests.

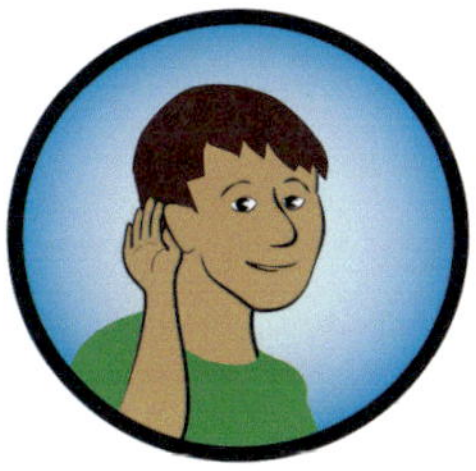

2. **LISTEN**—Carefully listen to what the other person is talking about so you can know what the topic is. "Capture" a detail or two that you can ask about when it is your turn. By doing your best to use your **power** to concentrate on the other person's topic, you are showing that you **care** about him or her.

3. **MAKE COMMENTS AND ASK QUESTIONS**—Show the other person you are **respectful** and **cooperative** by making comments and asking questions about something the other person said.

4. **KEEP TRACK OF THE TOPICS THAT THE OTHER PERSON LIKES TO TALK ABOUT SO YOU CAN INITIATE CONVERSATIONS ABOUT THAT TOPIC!**—You can use the **CARING CONVERSATION UPDATE SHEET** for each Team member with whom you will be having conversations. By continuing to add to this sheet you will have an updated log that will help you remember the different topics that your conversation partner thinks are important. By initiating asking about these topics, it will show your conversation partner that you care enough to remember what is interesting and important to them.

The more you practice having these conversations, the easier it will be to show your growing conversation **power**.

Wise Action Tool #35

BUILDING MY CONVERSATION POWER BY PAYING ATTENTION, ASKING QUESTIONS & TAKING NOTES

1A. I AM TALKING TO ______________________________ Date ____________________________

1B. I CHOOSE A TOPIC: This is a topic that I think this person would like to talk about today: _______

____

2. I ASK A QUESTION: I ask a question to learn something new about the topic:

How is ____?

or *Tell me what's new with* ____

3. I LISTEN AND TAKE NOTES: I use my **power** to listen carefully and write down an important detail about what was said: ____

____

4. I MAKE A COMMENT: (*Wow! That's interesting! That's great! Sounds good! Too bad.*) _______

____

5. I ASK A RELATED QUESTION: I ask another question about what the person just said:

How do you feel about ____?

Can you tell me more about ____?

What _________________? *Where* ___________________? *Why* ___________________?

6. I LISTEN AND TAKE NOTES: I use my **power** to listen carefully and write down an important detail about what was said: ____

____

7. I MAKE A FINAL COMMENT THAT SHOWS I WAS LISTENING TO WHAT THE PERSON SAID:
I politely end the conversation by saying one or more of the following:

That's very interesting! Thanks for telling me about ______________________________

I'm glad that ____

or I'm sorry that ____

and I hope that ____

(When we are done talking, I can draw a detailed picture to help me remember what my conversation partner said about this topic.)

Wise Action Tool #36

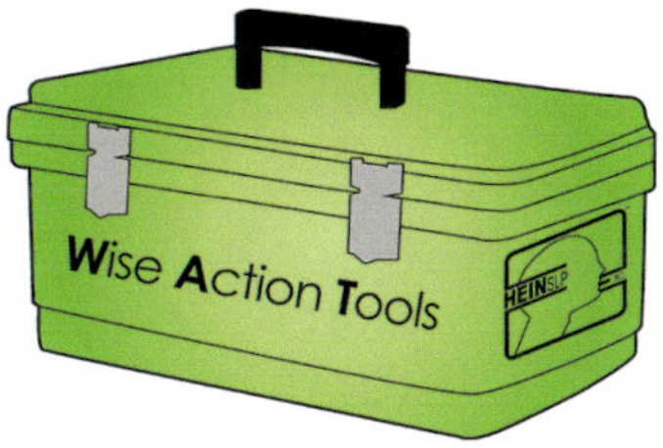

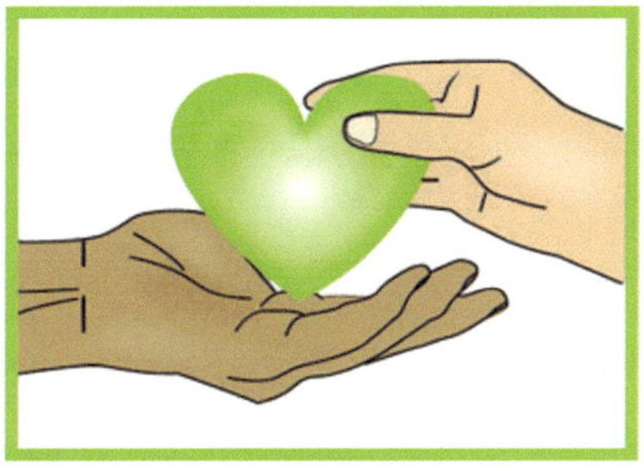

TOPICS FOR CARING CONVERSATIONS

I care about these people, so I keep track of the topics they care about. I can show I care by talking about these topics in my conversations with them.

Person I Care About	This Person Cares About These Topics

Wise Action Tool #37

Wise Action Tools

VOICE VOLUME CHART

WAY TOO LOUD!!!
MEDIUM LOUD
A LITTLE TOO LOUD
Just Right For The Room & The People
A little too soft
much too soft to be heard
I can't hear you!!

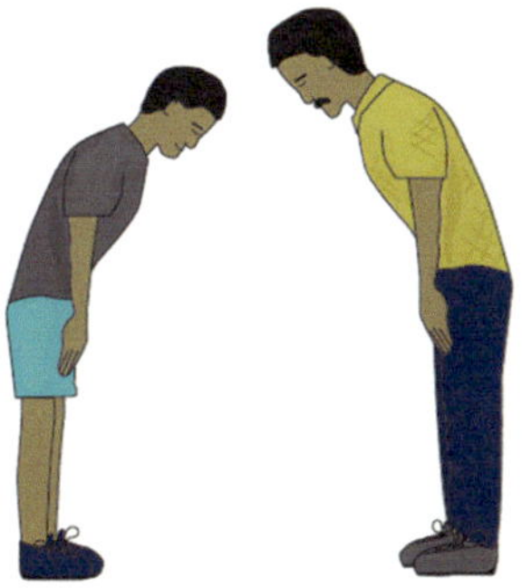

Wise Action Tool #38

HEIN CONVERSATIONAL RATING SCALE

I have to think about:

- my choice of topic and if it is appropriate for my audience
- my choice of words and if they are appropriate for my audience
- my tone of voice
- my audience
- how much humor/teasing I can safely use with my audience and still be taken seriously when needed

G = General Audiences—What I say would be OK with Grandma or the school principal. I am on topic and am not saying anything odd, strange, mean, disgusting, or violent. No swear words are used at all. I get a lot of social points for being able to control my topic and my words. I am considered mature.

PG = Possible Guidance needed—What I want to say may be slightly funny or sarcastic. I need to know if my audience will appreciate my topic and words without my losing social points. With this style, I might be considered immature.

R = Restricted—The topic and word choice would offend most people. I can use this language only at special times with people who would appreciate my odd, strange, mean, disgusting, or violent topics. If I use this language in class or public, I will get in trouble and lose many social points. People will not trust that I can control myself and I will lose privileges and responsibilities. I should avoid saying things that are really off topic because people will consider them R-rated and will not want to have conversations with me in the future.

X = eXtremely Limited—These topics and words are so inappropriate, strange, odd, violent, disgusting, or mean that they really should not be said out loud. I should limit even thinking about these topics or words. Most people will be extremely offended, upset, or worried if they hear these words or topics, and I will get in serious trouble and lose all my social points.

Wise Action Tool #39

CONNECTION DIRECTION TRACKER

AM I MOVING FORWARD, OR BACKWARD, WITH MY TEAM?

Take a step forward to connect →

I took steps to *disconnect* from other people.	-4	-3	-2	-1	0	+1	+2	+3	+4	I took steps to make positive civilized connections with other people.

← Take a step backward to disconnect

Wise Action Tool #40

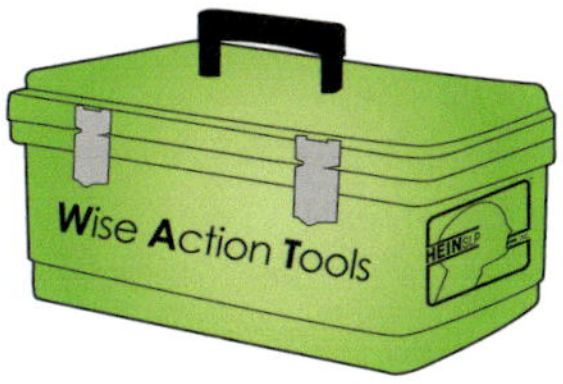

NAME MIXED FEELINGS AND THINK OF ACTION CONSEQUENCES

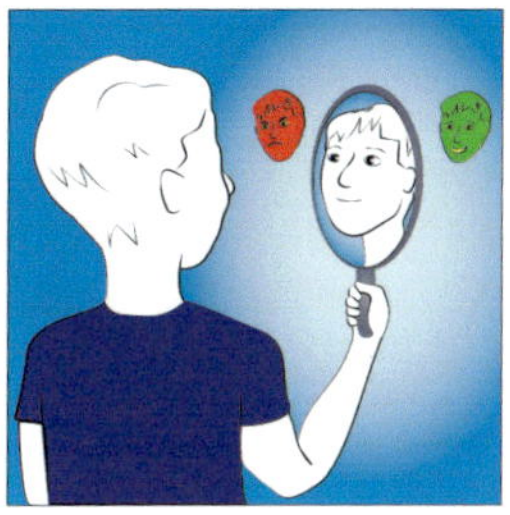

1. I put on my brakes to get **self-control**!
2. I Think First!
3. I name my **mixed** feelings.
4. I think of the **positive** & **negative** consequences of acting upon **outside** and **inside** feelings.
5. I think about how I help myself and my Team when I act upon my **positive outside** feelings instead of my **negative inside** feelings.

1. Name my inside negative feelings: What name can I give to these negative feelings? ________________________	1. Name my possible outside **positive** feelings: What name can I give to these **positive** feelings? ________________________
2. Why could I be feeling these feelings? ________________________ ________________________	2. Why could I be feeling these feelings? ________________________ ________________________
3. Negative consequences of showing my negative feelings: What would the negative consequences be if I acted upon these negative feelings by acting **R.E.D.**? ________________________ ________________________ ________________________	3. **Positive** consequences of showing my **positive** feelings: What would the **positive** consequences be if I acted upon these **positive** feelings by acting **G.R.E.E.N.**? ________________________ ________________________ ________________________
4. I take action to find ways to weaken these negative feelings to *avoid* acting **R.E.D.**	4. I work to strengthen these **positive** feelings so it is easier to take **G.R.E.E.N.** action with my Team?

Wise Action Tool #41

SHOW POSITIVE OUTSIDE ACTION CONTROL!

Draw POSITIVE OUTSIDE feelings, words, and actions

Draw NEGATIVE INSIDE feelings and actions

Wise Action Tool #42

COOPERATIVE CONVERSATION INGREDIENTS CHECKLIST

Name ______________________________ Date ____________________

Think about the ingredients needed in a Cooperative Conversation. Mark this checklist to show whether Persons #1 and #2 have included those ingredients.

Situation Topic: ____

____

Common Team Goal ____

____

Ingredients for a Cooperative Conversation	Name of Person #1: ______	Name of Person #2: ______	Did both people work **cooperatively**?
1. Calmly and respectfully *tell* what each person needs.	Did this person calmly and respecttfully use words to say what was needed? yes no	Did this person calmly and respecttfully use words to say what was needed? yes no	Did both people have a chance to *tell* what they wanted or needed? yes no
2. Respectfully and patiently listen to what each person needs.	Did this person respectfully and patiently listen to what the other person needed? yes no	Did this person respectfully and patiently listen to what the other person needed? yes no	Did both people listen to find out what the other person wanted or needed? yes no
3. Respectfully and patiently use words to *share ideas, making a plan* to meet *both* people's needs. Both people win!	Did this person say some-thing to help the other person feel that their needs will be met? yes no	Did this person say some-thing to help the other person feel that their needs will be met? yes no	Did both pople work together to flexibly find a way to meet each other's needs? yes no

Are all ingredients included? yes no

If not, circle the ingredients to add to make the next conversation more cooperative.

Wise Action Tool #43

I ACCEPT CONSTRUCTIVE FEEDBACK IN THESE AREAS

I show that I am more **easygoing** and **open-minded** when I accept **constructive feedback** in many of these areas. I can add more of these areas as I become more comfortable about accepting feedback from others. Using feedback from others helps me reach my **goals**. As of the date noted below, I accept **constructive feedback** in these areas:

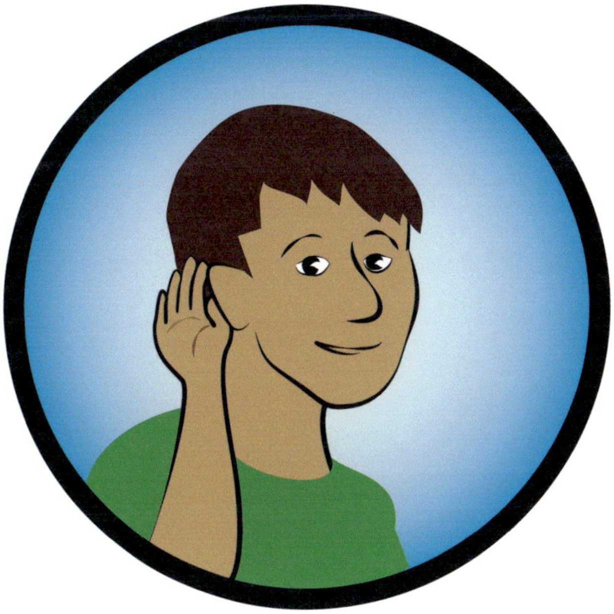

Editing my writing ______________

Playing sports ____________

Getting along with others ________

Managing my time ___________

Studying or doing my homework _____

Doing my chores _______________

Taking care of my grooming ____________

Solving problems ____________

Thinking before I act ________

Using the right tone of voice_____________

Choosing the right words ______________

Respectfully asking for help ______________________

Getting along with friends _____________________

Showing empathy for others _____________________

Name ____________________________________ Date ______________________

Wise Action Tool #44

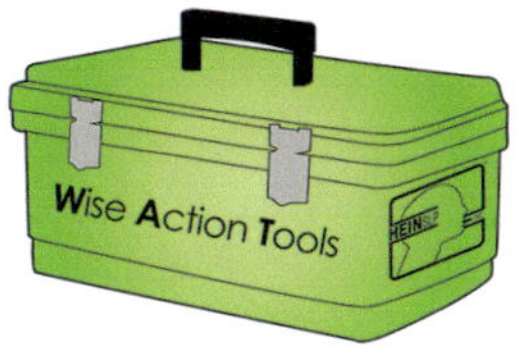

WORKSHEET FOR MAKING A G.R.E.E.N. TEAM COMPROMISE

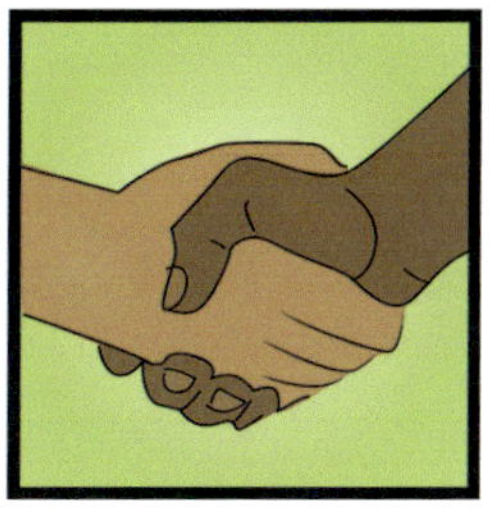

Here is the situation that needs a Team compromise:

____

____

____

Our Shared G.R.E.E.N. Compromise:

This is the G.R.E.E.N. compromise we have made together.

We both get some needs met so we can both move forward.

If I ____

____

then you ____

____

If you ____

____

then I ____

____

Wise Action Tool #45

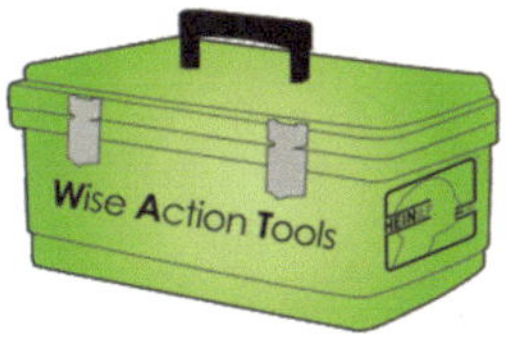

CHARTING HOW MUCH HELP I NEED TODAY

____

TODAY'S DATE

I Keep track of how much help I need to do things. This helps me and others know what I can do by myself and what things I can do with help. I can have **Personal Goals** to build my skills and work hard to move things over to the left on this chart. I can work to move things from the list of things I can't do, to the list of things I can do with help, and then to the list of things I can do by myself. First, I will write on this chart how much help I need doing things today! Then I will see how much progress I have made the next time I fill out this chart.

Things I can do well **by myself**	Things I can do well **if I get some help**	Things I **can't do** right now

My name ____

Wise Action Tool #46

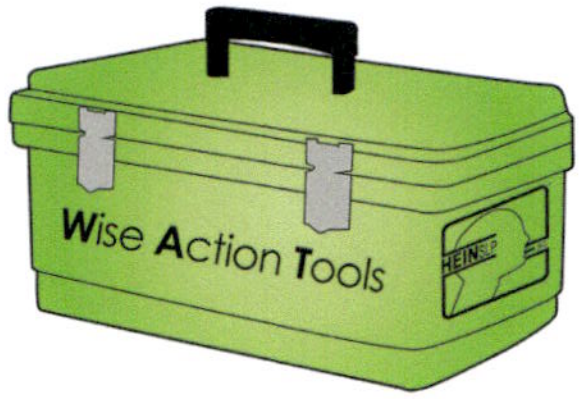

LESSON LOG FOR WHAT I AM LEARNING

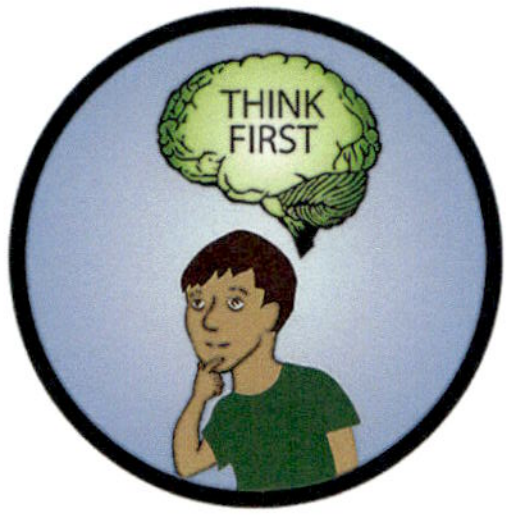

Date	Main Idea of What I Did and Learned Today

Wise Action Tool #47

GROWING G.R.E.E.N. CERTIFICATE

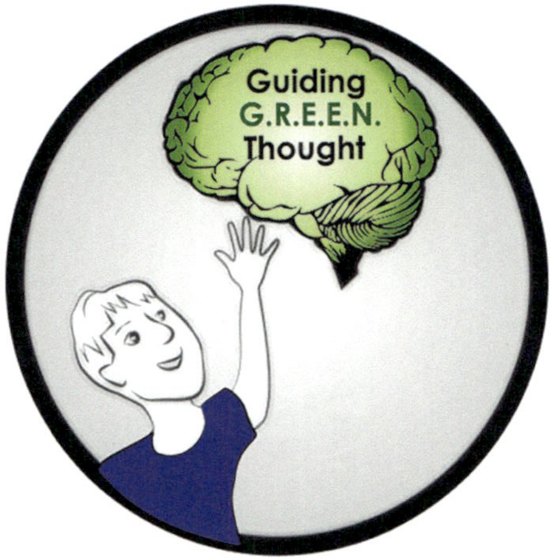

______________________________ has been:

☐ Thoughtful	☐ Respectful
☐ Positive	☐ Kind
☐ Open-Minded	☐ Cooperative

Presented by __________________ Date _____________

Wise Action Tool #48

Made in the USA
Las Vegas, NV
03 November 2026

57423446R00067